MUSCLE FOR LIFE
FITNESS JOURNAL

MUSCLE FOR LIFE FITNESS JOURNAL

A 12-Month Program for Transforming
Your Body and Health at Any Age

MICHAEL MATTHEWS

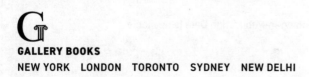

GALLERY BOOKS

NEW YORK   LONDON   TORONTO   SYDNEY   NEW DELHI

Gallery Books
An Imprint of Simon & Schuster, LLC
1230 Avenue of the Americas
New York, NY 10020

This publication contains the opinions and ideas of its author. It is intended to provide helpful and informative material on the subjects addressed in the publication. It is sold with the understanding that the author and publisher are not engaged in rendering medical, health, or any other kind of personal professional services in the book. The reader should consult his or her medical, health, or other competent professional before adopting any of the suggestions in this book or drawing inferences from it.

The author and publisher specifically disclaim all responsibility for any liability, loss, or risk, personal or otherwise, which is incurred as a consequence, directly or indirectly, of the use and application of any of the contents of this book.

First Gallery Books trade paperback edition December 2024

GALLERY BOOKS and colophon are registered trademarks of Simon & Schuster, LLC

Simon & Schuster: Celebrating 100 Years of Publishing in 2024

For information about special discounts for bulk purchases, please contact Simon & Schuster Special Sales at 1-866-506-1949 or business@simonandschuster.com.

The Simon & Schuster Speakers Bureau can bring authors to your live event. For more information or to book an event, contact the Simon & Schuster Speakers Bureau at 1-866-248-3049 or visit our website at www.simonspeakers.com.

Interior design by Matt Ryan

Printed and bound by CPI (UK) Ltd, Croydon CR0 4YY

10 9 8 7 6 5 4 3 2

Library of Congress Cataloging-in-Publication Data is available.

ISBN 978-1-6680-3486-6

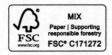

Thank you to everyone who helped me create this book, including Mary and Armi, who are the ace up my sleeve; Rebecca, who made a special effort to champion and nurture this project; Rick, who guided me with integrity and grace; and everyone else who helped get this work into your hands.

And last but foremost, thank *you* for supporting my work and giving me the opportunity to help you transform your body and health. Let's get the bit between your teeth, and before you know it, you're going to look back and think, "Wow, all of those little improvements really did add up."

CONTENTS

AUTHOR'S NOTE

> "It's from the champions of
> the impossible, rather than
> from slaves of the possible,
> that evolution draws its
> creative force."
> —BARBARA WOOTTON

THANK YOU FOR CHOOSING THE *Muscle for Life Fitness Journal*. I hope you find this journal insightful, inspiring, and practical, and I hope it helps you build the fit, strong, and healthy body you really desire.

I want to make sure that you get as much value from this journal as possible, so I've put together a number of additional free resources to help you, including:

- All of the workouts in this journal (plus bonus workouts), neatly laid out and provided in several digital formats, including PDF, Excel, and Google Sheets
- Links to form demonstration videos for all *Muscle for Life* exercises
- Twenty *Muscle for Life* meal plans that make losing fat and gaining lean muscle as simple as possible
- My product recommendations for workout equipment, gear, and gadgets like home gym equipment, shoes, gloves, straps, and more
- A list of my favorite tools for getting and staying motivated and on track inside and outside of the gym
- A list of my all-time favorite fitness books
- And more

To get instant access to all of those free bonuses (plus a few additional surprise gifts), go here now:

» www.mfljournal.com/bonus

FITNESS ISN'T EVERYTHING.

BUT EVERYTHING IS HARDER IF YOU AREN'T FIT.

1 HOW TO USE THIS JOURNAL

> **"Death is nothing, but to live
> defeated is to die every day."**
>
> —NAPOLEON BONAPARTE

SIR WILLIAM THOMSON (ALSO KNOWN as Lord Kelvin, namesake of the Kelvin temperature scale used by researchers) was a brilliant nineteenth-century physicist, and his insight on the importance of measuring applies to many things in life, including exercise and diet. Only when you can measure your progress (or lack thereof) and express it in real numbers, he said, can you know whether you're headed in the right direction. If you don't have any consistent, objective way to assess progress, however, you're working blind and hoping for the best. This is one of the major reasons so many people fail to achieve their fitness goals, and why I created this fitness journal.

Monitoring the wrong things—or monitoring the right things in the wrong way—can mislead you on your fitness journey and impede your progress. For example, many people use electronic devices or smartphone apps to estimate calories burned in workouts and track their body composition. Research shows that these gadgets and software are notoriously inaccurate. Similarly, while body weight is important to watch, daily fluctuations aren't important, so cursing or cheering them is counterproductive to long-term progress.

Tracking changes in body composition (e.g., weight, inches lost or gained, etc.) is a popular way of charting your progress, but tracking your strength training is just as important. Monitoring your strength training is the only way to ensure you're *progressively overloading* your muscles (increasing the amount of muscular tension generated during training over time), which is the only way to consistently gain muscle and strength. At first your strength will shoot up by leaps and bounds, but in time progress will slow, and the details get hazy if you don't have a training journal. You won't remember what you did in your previous workouts and thus won't know if your strength is going up or down.

Remember that as you become more experienced, a successful workout is one where you beat your last performance by even a little—perhaps a rep or two with the same weight on just one exercise. For example, if you know your first hard set of squats in your previous lower-body workout was 135 pounds for 8 reps, in this next workout all you should have on your mind is hitting 9 or 10 reps with that same weight.

Tracking your training also makes it more exciting—you get to watch hard data change for the better and, as time passes, review old records and bask in how far you've come and how committed you are to your goals.

Above all, this fitness journal is for doing and tracking *Muscle for Life* workouts, so it contains one year's worth of training for men and women divided into three training phases that build on each other: Phase One (the first four months), Phase Two (the next four months), and Phase Three (the final four months). You'll learn more about the phases and workouts in chapter 3, including how to determine where to start, how to do the workouts, how to progress from one phase to the next, and how to avoid injury.

What's more, after each phase of training, we'll engage in productive reflection on how it went, how you're doing, and how we can make the next month even better. Remember to check in after you complete each four-week training block for a short reflection and, if needed, adjustment to your regimen.

Before you learn about and launch into the workouts, however, let's review the exercises you'll be doing in them.

SOMETIMES THE BEST WORKOUTS ARE THE ONES YOU LEAST WANT TO DO.

2 THE *MUSCLE FOR LIFE EXERCISES*

> **"If you don't make time for your wellness, you will be forced to make time for your illness."**
> —JOYCE SUNADA

OF ALL THE STRENGTH TRAINING exercises you can do, a few dozen stand head and shoulders above the rest in terms of ease of execution, measurable effects, and overall impact. And of those, a handful are the real stars.

This is great news for us because it means we can disregard most of what we see people doing in magazines, on social media, and at the gym, and focus instead on getting strong on a short list of exercises.

In fact, constantly changing exercises to challenge your body in new ways is a poor strength training strategy. The more often you make a switch, the harder it is to become proficient at any of the exercises you're doing, and this slows your progress. If you stick with a relatively small selection of highly effective exercises that allow you to safely overload your muscles, however, you can get fit and strong faster than you ever thought possible.

In this chapter, I'll share those superior exercises with you, separated into two categories:

1. Primary exercises
2. Accessory exercises

Primary exercises will be responsible for the lion's share of your results because they train (and develop) the most muscle mass and produce the most whole-body strength. As effective as the primary exercises are, however, some muscles are particularly stubborn and slow to respond to training, and others aren't adequately trained by primary exercises alone. We'll use *accessory exercises* to address these issues—further training muscle groups that need more stimulation than primary exercises alone can provide—and also to help prevent and correct muscle imbalances and weaknesses that can limit your progress on your primary exercises.

The exercises will be divided into pushing, pulling, and squatting movements, and the primary exercises will be designated beginner, intermediate, or advanced (there isn't a big enough difference in difficulty between the accessory exercises to require the same distinctions).

The following chart shows the exercises included in the *Muscle for Life* program classified by type and difficulty. No matter where you begin, you are working toward the ultimate goal of mastering the advanced exercises, which may take a year or longer depending on your current level of fitness.

	PUSHING EXERCISES	PULLING EXERCISES	SQUATTING EXERCISES
BEGINNER PRIMARY EXERCISES	Push-up	Bodyweight Row	Bodyweight Squat
	Machine Chest Press	Dumbbell Deadlift	Bodyweight Split Squat
	Machine Shoulder Press	One-Arm Dumbbell Row	Bodyweight Lunge
	Triceps Dip		Bodyweight Step-up
			Leg Press

	PUSHING EXERCISES	PULLING EXERCISES	SQUATTING EXERCISES
INTERMEDIATE PRIMARY EXERCISES	Dumbbell Bench Press	Trap-Bar Deadlift	Dumbbell Goblet Squat
	Incline Dumbbell Bench Press	Seated Cable Row	Dumbbell Lunge
	Seated Dumbbell Overhead Press		Dumbbell Split Squat
			Dumbbell Romanian Deadlift
ADVANCED PRIMARY EXERCISES	Barbell Bench Press	Barbell Deadlift	Barbell Back Squat
	Incline Barbell Bench Press	Chin-up	Barbell Romanian Deadlift
	Chest Dip	Pull-up	
ACCESSORIES	Cable Triceps Pushdown	Lat Pulldown	Leg Extension
	Dumbbell Triceps Overhead Press	Machine Row	Leg Curl
	Machine Cable Fly	Alternating Dumbbell Curl	Glute Bridge
		Cable Biceps Curl	

Although the lingo can make these movements sound formidable, you can rest assured that they're simple enough for anyone to pick up, regardless of their athletic aptitude. Also, to help you visualize each of the movements, I've included links to video demonstrations of them in the free bonus material that comes with this book (www.mfljournal.com/bonus).

ONE DAY, YOU'RE GOING TO LOOK BACK AND THINK,

"WOW, ALL OF THOSE LITTLE IMPROVEMENTS REALLY DID ADD UP."

3 | THE *MUSCLE FOR LIFE* PROGRAM

> **"You are what you do,
> not what you say you'll do."**
> —CARL JUNG

IN THIS CHAPTER, YOU'LL LEARN the key elements of the *Muscle for Life* program as well as simple solutions to issues that you might run into as you find your feet (like how heavy your weights should be, how you should warm up, and so on). Then we'll discuss cardiovascular exercise and how to incorporate it into your training regimen without overextending yourself.

THE *MUSCLE FOR LIFE* TRAINING PHASE

In *Muscle for Life*, a training phase is a seventeen-week block of training designed to increase strength and muscle size and definition. Every phase is separated into two parts:

1. HARD TRAINING. Each training phase begins with sixteen weeks of challenging workouts designed to increase strength and muscularity (followed by an assessment of your performance and progress).

2. DELOADING. Each training phase ends with one week of deloading to facilitate recovery.

This journal contains three training phases, and thus provides you with a year's worth of *Muscle for Life* workouts. What's more, the phases in this journal correspond to the three levels of difficulty discussed in *Muscle for Life*—beginner, intermediate, and advanced. Later we'll discuss how to determine which phase to start with and how to progress in your training.

THE *MUSCLE FOR LIFE* STRENGTH TRAINING ROUTINES

Whereas a training phase delineates the goals and duration of a training block, a training routine outlines what you'll do in that time to achieve those goals—how often you'll train and what you'll do in each workout.

The *Muscle for Life* program comprises three different workout routines for men and three for women: beginner (Phase One), intermediate (Phase Two), and advanced (Phase Three). All routines call for three workouts per week, and as most guys especially want to buff up their "beach muscles" and most gals want to tone up their gams and glutes, the men's programs emphasize upper-body training whereas the women's spotlight the lower body.

If you're female and seeking upper-body definition or a male who's after lower-body size and strength, however, simply follow the other routine.

As for the different phases, Phase One workouts are suitable for someone new to proper strength training. They use bodyweight exercises to introduce you to the foundational movement patterns (push, pull, and squat) that effectively and efficiently train all of the major muscle groups in your body.

The Phase Two workouts are intermediate in difficulty, graduating you from calisthenics to weight lifting. With these workouts, you'll build a bedrock of muscle and strength that will put you well on your way to your ideal physique.

The Phase Three workouts are the most challenging in the *Muscle for Life* program because they incorporate barbell exercises, which are the most demanding type of resistance training but also the most rewarding. With Phase Three, you'll have everything you need to achieve first-class strength, definition, and function.

If you're new to *Muscle for Life*–style strength training or haven't trained consistently in at least a year, start with Phase One. If you dally with strength training and meet the following strength standards, start with Phase Two.

MEN'S STRENGTH STANDARDS	WOMEN'S STRENGTH STANDARDS
1 set of 15 feet-elevated push-ups	1 set of 10 push-ups
1 set of 15 bodyweight rows*	1 set of 10 bodyweight rows*
1 set of 15 bodyweight squats	1 set of 15 bodyweight squats

*With your body as close to parallel with the ground as possible (the most difficult variation of the exercise).

If you're an experienced trainee who meets or exceeds the following strength standards, start with Phase Three:

- **DUMBBELL BENCH PRESS:** 25 percent of your body weight (both dumbbells combined) for at least 1 set of 5 reps
- **TRAP-BAR DEADLIFT:** 75 percent of your body weight for at least 1 set of 5 reps
- **DUMBBELL GOBLET SQUAT:** 25 percent of your body weight for at least 1 set of 5 reps

Although the details of the workouts differ, all of the routines follow the same template: they entail three workouts per week, with one for the upper body and two for the lower body, or else two for the upper body and one for the lower body, depending on the routine. These workouts are labeled A or B (simply to differentiate them), with the upper-body training focused on pushing and pulling and the lower-body on squatting.

HOW TO DO *MUSCLE FOR LIFE* WORKOUTS

Most people prefer to do their strength training workouts on Monday, Wednesday, and Friday and take the weekends off, but you can work in your rest days however you'd like. The important thing is that you complete each of the workouts every seven days and in the order given. Here are some helpful considerations when creating your workout schedule:

- Try to evenly space your strength training workouts throughout the week.
- Try to include at least one day of no strength training between your strength training workouts.
- Many people, including myself, enjoy doing their strength training workouts during the week and keeping the weekends free for cardio and other activities.

When doing a workout, do the exercises in the order given, do warm-up sets when needed (see below), complete all *hard sets* (training sets taken close to failure) of one exercise before moving on to the next, and after each hard set, record the weight used and reps done.

Some people also like to record general details about how their workouts went as well as key factors that influenced their performance, such as diet, sleep, and general stress levels. For instance, they might note down that they slept well the night before and felt particularly strong in today's workout, or that they were short on calories the day before and noticed a slight decrease in energy in the gym.

Here's an example of how a completed workout might look:

MEN'S PHASE 1 STRENGTH TRAINING ROUTINE PHASE 1 · UPPER BODY A			
EXERCISES	SET 1	SET 2	SET 3
PUSH-UP	Bodyweight (BW) x 15	BW x 13	BW x 12
LAT PULLDOWN	45 x 14	45 x 13	45 x 11
MACHINE CHEST PRESS	40 x 12	35 x 15	35 x 14
BODYWEIGHT ROW	BW x 14	BW x 13	BW x 13

Simply recording everything you do isn't sufficient, though. You have to analyze the data to shape your training, and the easiest way to do that is to review previous sessions before repeating them. Then you can set targets for your next workouts.

Take the workout given above as an example. You did 13 reps in your second set of push-ups, nearing your goal of 15 reps. Next time, then, aim for 15 reps in your first set, 14 or 15 reps in the second set, and a minimum of 12 reps in your final set, surpassing your previous effort by at least one rep (progress!). And speaking of progress . . .

HOW TO PROGRESS IN *MUSCLE FOR LIFE* WORKOUTS

In *Muscle for Life*, you'll advance your fitness in two ways: by adding weight to the exercises and by increasing the difficulty of the exercises.

To add weight, you'll use a method called *double progression*, which involves working with a given weight until you can do a number of hard sets (usually 1, 2, or 3) in a row of a number of reps (usually the top of the rep range you're working in, like 15 in 12-to-15 reps). Once you've achieved your "progression target," you then add weight to the exercise (or upgrade to a more difficult exercise) and work with that new weight or exercise until reaching your progression target again. Here's how to implement double progression in *Muscle for Life*:

In Phase One training, in the case of a bodyweight exercise, switch to a harder exercise variation, and in the case of a dumbbell exercise, increase the total weight by 10 pounds (5 pounds per dumbbell) when you can do 3 hard sets in a row of 15 reps. And if you're just starting out and can't do 3 hard sets in a row of at least 10 reps of a bodyweight exercise, swap it for an easier variation.

So, let's say you're doing an upper-body workout, and you got 15 regular push-ups in your first hard set followed by 14 and 13 reps in the next 2 hard sets. You're not ready to progress yet (3 hard sets in a row of at least 15 reps), so you shouldn't change anything. A couple of weeks later, however, you get 15 reps in each of your 3 hard sets, which means you can start doing feet-elevated push-ups in your next upper-body workouts.

Or instead, maybe you got 10 regular push-ups in your first hard set and just 8 and 6 reps in the next 2 hard sets. You're not reaching the lower performance threshold for the exercise (10+ reps per hard set), so you should do knee push-ups instead until you get 3 hard sets in a row of at least 15 reps. Then you can return to regular push-ups (with enough strength to do at least 10 reps per hard set).

In Phase Two of the program, increase the weight on an exercise by 10 pounds (5 pounds per dumbbell) when you can do 3 hard sets in a row of 12 reps. And if you can't do 3 hard sets in a row of at least 10 reps on an exercise, the weight is too heavy, so reduce the load by 10 pounds (total), rest, and reassess. If you still can't do 3 hard sets in a row of at least 10 reps, reduce the weight further until you can, and continue working with that weight.

Another illustration: let's say you do 3 hard sets in a row of 12 reps on the trap-bar deadlift. What do you do? You got it—add 10 pounds to the bar (5 on either side) and continue until you can do 3 hard sets in a row of at least 12 reps (followed by another 10 pounds added to the bar).

In Phase Three's workouts, increase the weight by 10 pounds (5 pounds per dumbbell) when you can do 3 hard sets in a row of 10 reps. Reduce the weight if you can't do 3 hard sets in a row of at least 8 reps.

The second method of progression in *Muscle for Life* is proceeding from one phase to the next.

To graduate from Phase One to Two, you must fully complete at least one round of Phase One and meet the strength standards you learned a moment ago: if you're a man, you must be able to do 1 set each of at least 15 feet-elevated push-ups, bodyweight rows, and bodyweight squats; and if you're a woman, at least 1 set each of 10 push-ups and bodyweight rows and 1 set of 15 bodyweight squats.

To graduate from Phase Two to Three, you must fully complete at least one round of Phase Two and be able to dumbbell bench press 25 percent of your body weight for at least 1 set of 5 reps, trap-bar deadlift 75 percent of your body weight for at least 1 set of 5 reps, and dumbbell goblet squat 25 percent of your body weight for at least 1 set of 5 reps.

Now, this journal provides you with four months of Phase One workouts, four months of Phase Two workouts, and four months of Phase Three workouts. What should you do if, after four months of training, you're not ready for the next phase? Simply restart the phase you just completed, and by the end of your second round (if not sooner), you should be able to progress to the next one. And to track your workouts when repeating a phase, you can use the blank templates in the back of this book (provided for this purpose).

Thus, you should stick with Phase One until you a) complete it at least once, and b) qualify for Phase Two (even if that takes more than one round of Phase One), and stick with Phase Two until you've completed it at least once and qualify for Phase Three.

In the case of subsequent performances of a phase, once you qualify for the next phase, finish your current workouts for the week and begin your new ones the following week. Also, remember to deload when you would've on the easier routine. For example, if you switch from Phase One to Two on week fourteen of your first round of Phase One, you'd do two weeks of Phase Two training, deload, and carry on with your Phase Two workouts.

Finally, there are several other factors discussed in more detail in *Muscle for Life* that are vital to your long-term progress on the program, including:

- On bodyweight exercises, end hard sets at the point where you're 1 rep shy of muscle failure (you'll fail to complete the next rep).
- On machine, dumbbell, and barbell exercises, end hard sets at the point where you're 2 to 3 reps shy of muscle failure (you can perform 1 to 2 more reps before failing).
- Always use a full range of motion (don't do partial reps).
- Don't use gravity or momentum during sets. Always feel like you're using your muscles to control your body and the weight.
- Don't skip the warm-up sets. They boost performance and reduce the risk of injury.
- If something feels off or painful while you're working out, take a breather for a couple of minutes, and give it another shot. If it's still not feeling right on the second try, swap it out for a different exercise that feels okay, and come back to the sticky one in your next session to see how it goes. If it's still bugging you, trade it out for something else again and steer clear of the bothersome exercise until it feels fine.

Avoid pushing for gains by sacrificing proper form or piling on the plates before you're ready to handle them. Slow and steady is the aim of the game. For example, if you're just starting out with resistance training and you're able to bump up the weight on most of your exercises every week or two for the first few months, you're making good. And once you've got more experience under your belt, even adding a single rep per week on your toughest lifts (and therefore increasing the weight every few weeks) is nothing to sniff at.

IT'S SHOCKING HOW MANY WORRIES, SORROWS, AND DIFFICULTIES SIMPLY DISAPPEAR AFTER A WEEK OF GOOD SLEEP, NUTRITION, AND EXERCISE.

4 THE *MUSCLE FOR LIFE* WORKOUTS

> **"The best six doctors
> anywhere and no one can deny it,
> are sunshine, water, rest,
> and air, exercise and diet."**
> —WAYNE FIELDS

LAO TZU FAMOUSLY SAID THAT the journey of a thousand miles begins with a single step, and I'm excited that you're about to take *your* first step on my program. If you mostly stick to the plan (no need to even try to be perfect), you'll see dramatic improvements in your body in just the next few months. People won't believe their eyes. You might not, either!

You'll also realize just how simple improving your body composition really is. Never again will you struggle to gain muscle or lose fat, and never again will you fall prey to mainstream diet and exercise fads and hucksters. You'll know that you finally have "the way" to the body you've always wanted.

I have to warn you, though: the first eight to twelve weeks are always the hardest. I've worked with thousands of guys and gals over the years, and if someone is going to quit, it's usually within the first few months.

Sometimes it's because establishing new habits—even immediately beneficial ones—is difficult, sometimes it's because they succumb to peer pressure to go back to their old unhealthy ways, and sometimes it's because of unforeseen disruptions like sickness, stress, or other snags. However, the people who can stick through the first two or three months, come what may, often are the ones who never stop.

I want you to be one of these people. That's why I write books and articles, record podcasts and videos, and do everything else that I do. That's why I want you to promise me—and yourself—that you'll do whatever it takes to get through the first two phases of this challenge. You don't have to be perfect, of course—just good enough—and life may try to get in the way (in fact, it probably will), and you may have to get creative to find workarounds, but that's just part of the game.

The bottom line is this: if you make a firm decision to see it through, and then defend that decision against all odds, there's nothing that can stop you.

Can you make that promise right now? And can you write it down below to make it official?

_____

_____

_____

_____

_____

_____

_____

_____

_____

_____

_____

_____

_____

Now let's begin your first year of *Muscle for Life* by taking some measurements and pictures. I recommend that you do this every two weeks while following the program—but if that doesn't work for you, try to do it once at least every four weeks.

Take the following body measurements as described in chapter 13 of *Muscle for Life*:

- Date
- Weight
- Waist
- Chest
- Shoulders
- Upper legs
- Arms
- Calves

DATE	WEIGHT		WAIST	CHEST
	SHOULDERS	UPPER LEGS	ARMS	CALVES

You don't *have* to take all of these measurements if you don't want to, but you should at least record your weight and waist measurement.

Train hard and do well! I'll see you in a few months!

FOUR MONTHS OF WOMEN'S BEGINNER WORKOUTS

Women's Beginner Routine · Phase 1 · Week 1

WORKOUT 1: LOWER BODY A			
EXERCISES	**SETS** *TOTAL WEIGHT X REPS, E.G., 45 X 12*		
	SET 1	SET 2	SET 3
BODYWEIGHT SQUAT Warm-up and 3 hard sets of 12–15 reps	X	X	X
DUMBBELL DEADLIFT 3 hard sets of 12–15 reps	X	X	X
BODYWEIGHT SPLIT SQUAT 3 hard sets of 12–15 reps	X	X	X
TRICEPS DIP 3 hard sets of 12–15 reps	X	X	X

NOTES

_____

_____

_____

_____

_____

WORKOUT 2: UPPER BODY A			
EXERCISES	**SETS** *TOTAL WEIGHT X REPS, E.G., 45 X 12*		
	SET 1	SET 2	SET 3
PUSH-UP Warm-up and 3 hard sets of 12–15 reps	X	X	X
LAT PULLDOWN 3 hard sets of 12–15 reps	X	X	X

EXERCISES	SET 1	SET 2	SET 3
MACHINE CHEST PRESS 3 hard sets of 12–15 reps	X	X	X
BODYWEIGHT ROW 3 hard sets of 12–15 reps	X	X	X

NOTES

_____

_____

_____

_____

WORKOUT 3: LOWER BODY B			
EXERCISES	**SETS** _TOTAL WEIGHT X REPS, E.G., 45 X 12_		
	SET 1	SET 2	SET 3
DUMBBELL DEADLIFT Warm-up and 3 hard sets of 12–15 reps	X	X	X
BODYWEIGHT LUNGE (IN-PLACE) 3 hard sets of 12–15 reps	X	X	X
LEG PRESS 3 hard sets of 12–15 reps	X	X	X
LEG CURL (LYING OR SEATED) 3 hard sets of 12–15 reps	X	X	X

NOTES

_____

_____

_____

_____

Women's Beginner Routine · Phase 1 · Week 2

WORKOUT 1: LOWER BODY A

EXERCISES	SETS TOTAL WEIGHT X REPS, E.G., 45 X 12		
	SET 1	SET 2	SET 3
BODYWEIGHT SQUAT Warm-up and 3 hard sets of 12–15 reps	X	X	X
DUMBBELL DEADLIFT 3 hard sets of 12–15 reps	X	X	X
BODYWEIGHT SPLIT SQUAT 3 hard sets of 12–15 reps	X	X	X
TRICEPS DIP 3 hard sets of 12–15 reps	X	X	X

NOTES

_____

_____

_____

_____

_____

_____

WORKOUT 2: UPPER BODY A

EXERCISES	SETS TOTAL WEIGHT X REPS, E.G., 45 X 12		
	SET 1	SET 2	SET 3
PUSH-UP Warm-up and 3 hard sets of 12–15 reps	X	X	X
LAT PULLDOWN 3 hard sets of 12–15 reps	X	X	X

MICHAEL MATTHEWS

EXERCISES	SET 1	SET 2	SET 3
MACHINE CHEST PRESS 3 hard sets of 12–15 reps	X	X	X
BODYWEIGHT ROW 3 hard sets of 12–15 reps	X	X	X

NOTES

_____

_____

_____

_____

_____

WORKOUT 3: LOWER BODY B			
EXERCISES	**SETS** _TOTAL WEIGHT X REPS, E.G., 45 X 12_		
	SET 1	SET 2	SET 3
DUMBBELL DEADLIFT Warm-up and 3 hard sets of 12–15 reps	X	X	X
BODYWEIGHT LUNGE (IN-PLACE) 3 hard sets of 12–15 reps	X	X	X
LEG PRESS 3 hard sets of 12–15 reps	X	X	X
LEG CURL (LYING OR SEATED) 3 hard sets of 12–15 reps	X	X	X

NOTES

_____

_____

_____

_____

_____

Women's Beginner Routine · Phase 1 · Week 3

WORKOUT 1: LOWER BODY A

EXERCISES	SETS *TOTAL WEIGHT X REPS, E.G., 45 X 12*		
	SET 1	SET 2	SET 3
BODYWEIGHT SQUAT Warm-up and 3 hard sets of 12–15 reps	X	X	X
DUMBBELL DEADLIFT 3 hard sets of 12–15 reps	X	X	X
BODYWEIGHT SPLIT SQUAT 3 hard sets of 12–15 reps	X	X	X
TRICEPS DIP 3 hard sets of 12–15 reps	X	X	X

NOTES

_____

_____

_____

_____

_____

_____

_____

WORKOUT 2: UPPER BODY A

EXERCISES	SETS *TOTAL WEIGHT X REPS, E.G., 45 X 12*		
	SET 1	SET 2	SET 3
PUSH-UP Warm-up and 3 hard sets of 12–15 reps	X	X	X
LAT PULLDOWN 3 hard sets of 12–15 reps	X	X	X

EXERCISES	SET 1	SET 2	SET 3
MACHINE CHEST PRESS 3 hard sets of 12–15 reps	X	X	X
BODYWEIGHT ROW 3 hard sets of 12–15 reps	X	X	X

NOTES

WORKOUT 3: LOWER BODY B

EXERCISES	SETS *TOTAL WEIGHT X REPS, E.G., 45 X 12*		
	SET 1	SET 2	SET 3
DUMBBELL DEADLIFT Warm-up and 3 hard sets of 12–15 reps	X	X	X
BODYWEIGHT LUNGE (IN-PLACE) 3 hard sets of 12–15 reps	X	X	X
LEG PRESS 3 hard sets of 12–15 reps	X	X	X
LEG CURL (LYING OR SEATED) 3 hard sets of 12–15 reps	X	X	X

NOTES

Women's Beginner Routine · Phase 1 · Week 4

WORKOUT 1: LOWER BODY A			
EXERCISES	**SETS** *TOTAL WEIGHT X REPS, E.G., 45 X 12*		
	SET 1	**SET 2**	**SET 3**
BODYWEIGHT SQUAT Warm-up and 3 hard sets of 12–15 reps	X	X	X
DUMBBELL DEADLIFT 3 hard sets of 12–15 reps	X	X	X
BODYWEIGHT SPLIT SQUAT 3 hard sets of 12–15 reps	X	X	X
TRICEPS DIP 3 hard sets of 12–15 reps	X	X	X

NOTES

_____

_____

_____

_____

_____

_____

WORKOUT 2: UPPER BODY A			
EXERCISES	**SETS** *TOTAL WEIGHT X REPS, E.G., 45 X 12*		
	SET 1	**SET 2**	**SET 3**
PUSH-UP Warm-up and 3 hard sets of 12–15 reps	X	X	X
LAT PULLDOWN 3 hard sets of 12–15 reps	X	X	X

EXERCISES	SET 1	SET 2	SET 3
MACHINE CHEST PRESS 3 hard sets of 12–15 reps	X	X	X
BODYWEIGHT ROW 3 hard sets of 12–15 reps	X	X	X

NOTES

_____

_____

_____

_____

WORKOUT 3: LOWER BODY B

EXERCISES	SETS *TOTAL WEIGHT X REPS, E.G., 45 X 12*		
	SET 1	SET 2	SET 3
DUMBBELL DEADLIFT Warm-up and 3 hard sets of 12–15 reps	X	X	X
BODYWEIGHT LUNGE (IN-PLACE) 3 hard sets of 12–15 reps	X	X	X
LEG PRESS 3 hard sets of 12–15 reps	X	X	X
LEG CURL (LYING OR SEATED) 3 hard sets of 12–15 reps	X	X	X

NOTES

_____

_____

_____

_____

Women's Beginner Routine · Phase 1 · Week 5

WORKOUT 1: LOWER BODY A			
EXERCISES	**SETS** *TOTAL WEIGHT X REPS, E.G., 45 X 12*		
	SET 1	**SET 2**	**SET 3**
BODYWEIGHT SQUAT Warm-up and 3 hard sets of 12–15 reps	X	X	X
DUMBBELL DEADLIFT 3 hard sets of 12–15 reps	X	X	X
BODYWEIGHT SPLIT SQUAT 3 hard sets of 12–15 reps	X	X	X
TRICEPS DIP 3 hard sets of 12–15 reps	X	X	X

NOTES

_____

_____

_____

_____

_____

_____

_____

WORKOUT 2: UPPER BODY A			
EXERCISES	**SETS** *TOTAL WEIGHT X REPS, E.G., 45 X 12*		
	SET 1	**SET 2**	**SET 3**
PUSH-UP Warm-up and 3 hard sets of 12–15 reps	X	X	X
LAT PULLDOWN 3 hard sets of 12–15 reps	X	X	X

EXERCISES	SET 1	SET 2	SET 3
MACHINE CHEST PRESS 3 hard sets of 12–15 reps	X	X	X
BODYWEIGHT ROW 3 hard sets of 12–15 reps	X	X	X

NOTES

_____
_____
_____
_____

WORKOUT 3: LOWER BODY B

EXERCISES	SETS _TOTAL WEIGHT X REPS, E.G., 45 X 12_		
	SET 1	SET 2	SET 3
DUMBBELL DEADLIFT Warm-up and 3 hard sets of 12–15 reps	X	X	X
BODYWEIGHT LUNGE (IN-PLACE) 3 hard sets of 12–15 reps	X	X	X
LEG PRESS 3 hard sets of 12–15 reps	X	X	X
LEG CURL (LYING OR SEATED) 3 hard sets of 12–15 reps	X	X	X

NOTES

_____
_____
_____
_____

Women's Beginner Routine · Phase 1 · Week 6

WORKOUT 1: LOWER BODY A

EXERCISES	SETS TOTAL WEIGHT X REPS, E.G., 45 X 12		
	SET 1	SET 2	SET 3
BODYWEIGHT SQUAT Warm-up and 3 hard sets of 12–15 reps	X	X	X
DUMBBELL DEADLIFT 3 hard sets of 12–15 reps	X	X	X
BODYWEIGHT SPLIT SQUAT 3 hard sets of 12–15 reps	X	X	X
TRICEPS DIP 3 hard sets of 12–15 reps	X	X	X

NOTES

_____

_____

_____

_____

_____

_____

_____

WORKOUT 2: UPPER BODY A

EXERCISES	SETS TOTAL WEIGHT X REPS, E.G., 45 X 12		
	SET 1	SET 2	SET 3
PUSH-UP Warm-up and 3 hard sets of 12–15 reps	X	X	X
LAT PULLDOWN 3 hard sets of 12–15 reps	X	X	X

EXERCISES	SET 1	SET 2	SET 3
MACHINE CHEST PRESS 3 hard sets of 12–15 reps	X	X	X
BODYWEIGHT ROW 3 hard sets of 12–15 reps	X	X	X

NOTES

_____

_____

_____

_____

WORKOUT 3: LOWER BODY B

EXERCISES	SETS _TOTAL WEIGHT X REPS, E.G., 45 X 12_		
	SET 1	SET 2	SET 3
DUMBBELL DEADLIFT Warm-up and 3 hard sets of 12–15 reps	X	X	X
BODYWEIGHT LUNGE (IN-PLACE) 3 hard sets of 12–15 reps	X	X	X
LEG PRESS 3 hard sets of 12–15 reps	X	X	X
LEG CURL (LYING OR SEATED) 3 hard sets of 12–15 reps	X	X	X

NOTES

_____

_____

_____

_____

Women's Beginner Routine · Phase 1 · Week 7

WORKOUT 1: LOWER BODY A			
EXERCISES	**SETS** *TOTAL WEIGHT X REPS, E.G., 45 X 12*		
	SET 1	**SET 2**	**SET 3**
BODYWEIGHT SQUAT Warm-up and 3 hard sets of 12–15 reps	X	X	X
DUMBBELL DEADLIFT 3 hard sets of 12–15 reps	X	X	X
BODYWEIGHT SPLIT SQUAT 3 hard sets of 12–15 reps	X	X	X
TRICEPS DIP 3 hard sets of 12–15 reps	X	X	X

NOTES

WORKOUT 2: UPPER BODY A			
EXERCISES	**SETS** *TOTAL WEIGHT X REPS, E.G., 45 X 12*		
	SET 1	**SET 2**	**SET 3**
PUSH-UP Warm-up and 3 hard sets of 12–15 reps	X	X	X
LAT PULLDOWN 3 hard sets of 12–15 reps	X	X	X

EXERCISES	SET 1	SET 2	SET 3
MACHINE CHEST PRESS 3 hard sets of 12–15 reps	X	X	X
BODYWEIGHT ROW 3 hard sets of 12–15 reps	X	X	X

NOTES

_____

_____

_____

_____

WORKOUT 3: LOWER BODY B			
EXERCISES	**SETS** _TOTAL WEIGHT X REPS, E.G., 45 X 12_		
	SET 1	SET 2	SET 3
DUMBBELL DEADLIFT Warm-up and 3 hard sets of 12–15 reps	X	X	X
BODYWEIGHT LUNGE (IN-PLACE) 3 hard sets of 12–15 reps	X	X	X
LEG PRESS 3 hard sets of 12–15 reps	X	X	X
LEG CURL (LYING OR SEATED) 3 hard sets of 12–15 reps	X	X	X

NOTES

_____

_____

_____

_____

Women's Beginner Routine · Phase 1 · Week 8

WORKOUT 1: LOWER BODY A			
EXERCISES	**SETS** *TOTAL WEIGHT X REPS, E.G., 45 X 12*		
	SET 1	**SET 2**	**SET 3**
BODYWEIGHT SQUAT Warm-up and 3 hard sets of 12–15 reps	X	X	X
DUMBBELL DEADLIFT 3 hard sets of 12–15 reps	X	X	X
BODYWEIGHT SPLIT SQUAT 3 hard sets of 12–15 reps	X	X	X
TRICEPS DIP 3 hard sets of 12–15 reps	X	X	X

NOTES

_____

_____

_____

_____

_____

_____

WORKOUT 2: UPPER BODY A			
EXERCISES	**SETS** *TOTAL WEIGHT X REPS, E.G., 45 X 12*		
	SET 1	**SET 2**	**SET 3**
PUSH-UP Warm-up and 3 hard sets of 12–15 reps	X	X	X
LAT PULLDOWN 3 hard sets of 12–15 reps	X	X	X

EXERCISES	SET 1	SET 2	SET 3
MACHINE CHEST PRESS 3 hard sets of 12–15 reps	X	X	X
BODYWEIGHT ROW 3 hard sets of 12–15 reps	X	X	X

NOTES

_____

_____

_____

_____

_____

WORKOUT 3: LOWER BODY B

EXERCISES	SETS *TOTAL WEIGHT X REPS, E.G., 45 X 12*		
	SET 1	SET 2	SET 3
DUMBBELL DEADLIFT Warm-up and 3 hard sets of 12–15 reps	X	X	X
BODYWEIGHT LUNGE (IN-PLACE) 3 hard sets of 12–15 reps	X	X	X
LEG PRESS 3 hard sets of 12–15 reps	X	X	X
LEG CURL (LYING OR SEATED) 3 hard sets of 12–15 reps	X	X	X

NOTES

_____

_____

_____

_____

_____

Women's Beginner Routine · Phase 1 · Week 9

WORKOUT 1: LOWER BODY A			
EXERCISES	**SETS** *TOTAL WEIGHT X REPS, E.G., 45 X 12*		
	SET 1	**SET 2**	**SET 3**
BODYWEIGHT LUNGE (WALKING) Warm-up and 3 hard sets of 12–15 reps	X	X	X
DUMBBELL DEADLIFT 3 hard sets of 12–15 reps	X	X	X
BODYWEIGHT SQUAT 3 hard sets of 12–15 reps	X	X	X
TRICEPS DIP 3 hard sets of 12–15 reps	X	X	X

NOTES

_____

_____

_____

_____

_____

_____

_____

WORKOUT 2: UPPER BODY A			
EXERCISES	**SETS** *TOTAL WEIGHT X REPS, E.G., 45 X 12*		
	SET 1	**SET 2**	**SET 3**
PUSH-UP Warm-up and 3 hard sets of 12–15 reps	X	X	X
ONE-ARM DUMBBELL ROW 3 hard sets of 12–15 reps	X	X	X

MICHAEL MATTHEWS

EXERCISES	SET 1	SET 2	SET 3
MACHINE SHOULDER PRESS 3 hard sets of 12–15 reps	X	X	X
BODYWEIGHT ROW 3 hard sets of 12–15 reps	X	X	X

NOTES

_____

_____

_____

_____

_____

WORKOUT 3: LOWER BODY B

EXERCISES	SETS _TOTAL WEIGHT X REPS, E.G., 45 X 12_		
	SET 1	SET 2	SET 3
DUMBBELL DEADLIFT Warm-up and 3 hard sets of 12–15 reps	X	X	X
BODYWEIGHT STEP-UP 3 hard sets of 12–15 reps	X	X	X
LEG EXTENSION 3 hard sets of 12–15 reps	X	X	X
GLUTE BRIDGE 3 hard sets of 12–15 reps	X	X	X

NOTES

_____

_____

_____

_____

_____

Women's Beginner Routine · Phase 1 · Week 10

WORKOUT 1: LOWER BODY A

EXERCISES	SETS *TOTAL WEIGHT X REPS, E.G., 45 X 12*		
	SET 1	SET 2	SET 3
BODYWEIGHT LUNGE (WALKING) Warm-up and 3 hard sets of 12–15 reps	X	X	X
DUMBBELL DEADLIFT 3 hard sets of 12–15 reps	X	X	X
BODYWEIGHT SQUAT 3 hard sets of 12–15 reps	X	X	X
TRICEPS DIP 3 hard sets of 12–15 reps	X	X	X

NOTES

WORKOUT 2: UPPER BODY A

EXERCISES	SETS *TOTAL WEIGHT X REPS, E.G., 45 X 12*		
	SET 1	SET 2	SET 3
PUSH-UP Warm-up and 3 hard sets of 12–15 reps	X	X	X
ONE-ARM DUMBBELL ROW 3 hard sets of 12–15 reps	X	X	X

EXERCISES	SET 1	SET 2	SET 3
MACHINE SHOULDER PRESS 3 hard sets of 12–15 reps	X	X	X
BODYWEIGHT ROW 3 hard sets of 12–15 reps	X	X	X

NOTES

_____

_____

_____

_____

_____

WORKOUT 3: LOWER BODY B

EXERCISES	SETS *TOTAL WEIGHT X REPS, E.G., 45 X 12*		
	SET 1	SET 2	SET 3
DUMBBELL DEADLIFT Warm-up and 3 hard sets of 12–15 reps	X	X	X
BODYWEIGHT STEP-UP 3 hard sets of 12–15 reps	X	X	X
LEG EXTENSION 3 hard sets of 12–15 reps	X	X	X
GLUTE BRIDGE 3 hard sets of 12–15 reps	X	X	X

NOTES

_____

_____

_____

_____

_____

Women's Beginner Routine · Phase 1 · Week 11

WORKOUT 1: LOWER BODY A			
EXERCISES	**SETS** *TOTAL WEIGHT X REPS, E.G., 45 X 12*		
	SET 1	**SET 2**	**SET 3**
BODYWEIGHT LUNGE (WALKING) Warm-up and 3 hard sets of 12–15 reps	X	X	X
DUMBBELL DEADLIFT 3 hard sets of 12–15 reps	X	X	X
BODYWEIGHT SQUAT 3 hard sets of 12–15 reps	X	X	X
TRICEPS DIP 3 hard sets of 12–15 reps	X	X	X

NOTES

_____

_____

_____

_____

_____

_____

_____

WORKOUT 2: UPPER BODY A			
EXERCISES	**SETS** *TOTAL WEIGHT X REPS, E.G., 45 X 12*		
	SET 1	**SET 2**	**SET 3**
PUSH-UP Warm-up and 3 hard sets of 12–15 reps	X	X	X
ONE-ARM DUMBBELL ROW 3 hard sets of 12–15 reps	X	X	X

EXERCISES	SET 1	SET 2	SET 3
MACHINE SHOULDER PRESS 3 hard sets of 12–15 reps	X	X	X
BODYWEIGHT ROW 3 hard sets of 12–15 reps	X	X	X

NOTES

WORKOUT 3: LOWER BODY B

EXERCISES	SETS *TOTAL WEIGHT X REPS, E.G., 45 X 12*		
	SET 1	SET 2	SET 3
DUMBBELL DEADLIFT Warm-up and 3 hard sets of 12–15 reps	X	X	X
BODYWEIGHT STEP-UP 3 hard sets of 12–15 reps	X	X	X
LEG EXTENSION 3 hard sets of 12–15 reps	X	X	X
GLUTE BRIDGE 3 hard sets of 12–15 reps	X	X	X

NOTES

Women's Beginner Routine · Phase 1 · Week 12

WORKOUT 1: LOWER BODY A

EXERCISES	SETS TOTAL WEIGHT X REPS, E.G., 45 X 12		
	SET 1	SET 2	SET 3
BODYWEIGHT LUNGE (WALKING) Warm-up and 3 hard sets of 12–15 reps	X	X	X
DUMBBELL DEADLIFT 3 hard sets of 12–15 reps	X	X	X
BODYWEIGHT SQUAT 3 hard sets of 12–15 reps	X	X	X
TRICEPS DIP 3 hard sets of 12–15 reps	X	X	X

NOTES

_____

_____

_____

_____

_____

_____

WORKOUT 2: UPPER BODY A

EXERCISES	SETS TOTAL WEIGHT X REPS, E.G., 45 X 12		
	SET 1	SET 2	SET 3
PUSH-UP Warm-up and 3 hard sets of 12–15 reps	X	X	X
ONE-ARM DUMBBELL ROW 3 hard sets of 12–15 reps	X	X	X

EXERCISES	SET 1	SET 2	SET 3
MACHINE SHOULDER PRESS 3 hard sets of 12–15 reps	X	X	X
BODYWEIGHT ROW 3 hard sets of 12–15 reps	X	X	X

NOTES

_____
_____
_____
_____
_____

WORKOUT 3: LOWER BODY B

EXERCISES	SETS _TOTAL WEIGHT X REPS, E.G., 45 X 12_		
	SET 1	SET 2	SET 3
DUMBBELL DEADLIFT Warm-up and 3 hard sets of 12–15 reps	X	X	X
BODYWEIGHT STEP-UP 3 hard sets of 12–15 reps	X	X	X
LEG EXTENSION 3 hard sets of 12–15 reps	X	X	X
GLUTE BRIDGE 3 hard sets of 12–15 reps	X	X	X

NOTES

_____
_____
_____
_____
_____

Women's Beginner Routine · Phase 1 · Week 13

WORKOUT 1: LOWER BODY A

EXERCISES	SETS TOTAL WEIGHT X REPS, E.G., 45 X 12		
	SET 1	SET 2	SET 3
BODYWEIGHT LUNGE (WALKING) Warm-up and 3 hard sets of 12–15 reps	X	X	X
DUMBBELL DEADLIFT 3 hard sets of 12–15 reps	X	X	X
BODYWEIGHT SQUAT 3 hard sets of 12–15 reps	X	X	X
TRICEPS DIP 3 hard sets of 12–15 reps	X	X	X

NOTES

_____

_____

_____

_____

_____

_____

_____

WORKOUT 2: UPPER BODY A

EXERCISES	SETS TOTAL WEIGHT X REPS, E.G., 45 X 12		
	SET 1	SET 2	SET 3
PUSH-UP Warm-up and 3 hard sets of 12–15 reps	X	X	X
ONE-ARM DUMBBELL ROW 3 hard sets of 12–15 reps	X	X	X

MICHAEL MATTHEWS

EXERCISES	SET 1	SET 2	SET 3
MACHINE SHOULDER PRESS 3 hard sets of 12–15 reps	X	X	X
BODYWEIGHT ROW 3 hard sets of 12–15 reps	X	X	X

NOTES

_____

_____

_____

_____

WORKOUT 3: LOWER BODY B

EXERCISES	SETS _TOTAL WEIGHT X REPS, E.G., 45 X 12_		
	SET 1	SET 2	SET 3
DUMBBELL DEADLIFT Warm-up and 3 hard sets of 12–15 reps	X	X	X
BODYWEIGHT STEP-UP 3 hard sets of 12–15 reps	X	X	X
LEG EXTENSION 3 hard sets of 12–15 reps	X	X	X
GLUTE BRIDGE 3 hard sets of 12–15 reps	X	X	X

NOTES

_____

_____

_____

_____

Women's Beginner Routine · Phase 1 · Week 14

WORKOUT 1: LOWER BODY A			
EXERCISES	**SETS** *TOTAL WEIGHT X REPS, E.G., 45 X 12*		
	SET 1	SET 2	SET 3
BODYWEIGHT LUNGE (WALKING) Warm-up and 3 hard sets of 12–15 reps	X	X	X
DUMBBELL DEADLIFT 3 hard sets of 12–15 reps	X	X	X
BODYWEIGHT SQUAT 3 hard sets of 12–15 reps	X	X	X
TRICEPS DIP 3 hard sets of 12–15 reps	X	X	X

NOTES

_____

_____

_____

_____

_____

_____

WORKOUT 2: UPPER BODY A			
EXERCISES	**SETS** *TOTAL WEIGHT X REPS, E.G., 45 X 12*		
	SET 1	SET 2	SET 3
PUSH-UP Warm-up and 3 hard sets of 12–15 reps	X	X	X
ONE-ARM DUMBBELL ROW 3 hard sets of 12–15 reps	X	X	X

MICHAEL MATTHEWS

EXERCISES	SET 1	SET 2	SET 3
MACHINE SHOULDER PRESS 3 hard sets of 12–15 reps	X	X	X
BODYWEIGHT ROW 3 hard sets of 12–15 reps	X	X	X

NOTES

_____

_____

_____

_____

WORKOUT 3: LOWER BODY B			
EXERCISES	**SETS** *TOTAL WEIGHT X REPS, E.G., 45 X 12*		
	SET 1	SET 2	SET 3
DUMBBELL DEADLIFT Warm-up and 3 hard sets of 12–15 reps	X	X	X
BODYWEIGHT STEP-UP 3 hard sets of 12–15 reps	X	X	X
LEG EXTENSION 3 hard sets of 12–15 reps	X	X	X
GLUTE BRIDGE 3 hard sets of 12–15 reps	X	X	X

NOTES

_____

_____

_____

_____

Women's Beginner Routine · Phase 1 · Week 15

WORKOUT 1: LOWER BODY A			
EXERCISES	**SETS** *TOTAL WEIGHT X REPS, E.G., 45 X 12*		
	SET 1	**SET 2**	**SET 3**
BODYWEIGHT LUNGE (WALKING) Warm-up and 3 hard sets of 12–15 reps	X	X	X
DUMBBELL DEADLIFT 3 hard sets of 12–15 reps	X	X	X
BODYWEIGHT SQUAT 3 hard sets of 12–15 reps	X	X	X
TRICEPS DIP 3 hard sets of 12–15 reps	X	X	X

NOTES

_____

_____

_____

_____

_____

_____

_____

WORKOUT 2: UPPER BODY A			
EXERCISES	**SETS** *TOTAL WEIGHT X REPS, E.G., 45 X 12*		
	SET 1	**SET 2**	**SET 3**
PUSH-UP Warm-up and 3 hard sets of 12–15 reps	X	X	X
ONE-ARM DUMBBELL ROW 3 hard sets of 12–15 reps	X	X	X

EXERCISES	SET 1	SET 2	SET 3
MACHINE SHOULDER PRESS 3 hard sets of 12–15 reps	X	X	X
BODYWEIGHT ROW 3 hard sets of 12–15 reps	X	X	X

NOTES

_____

_____

_____

_____

_____

WORKOUT 3: LOWER BODY B			
EXERCISES	**SETS** _TOTAL WEIGHT X REPS, E.G., 45 X 12_		
	SET 1	SET 2	SET 3
DUMBBELL DEADLIFT Warm-up and 3 hard sets of 12–15 reps	X	X	X
BODYWEIGHT STEP-UP 3 hard sets of 12–15 reps	X	X	X
LEG EXTENSION 3 hard sets of 12–15 reps	X	X	X
GLUTE BRIDGE 3 hard sets of 12–15 reps	X	X	X

NOTES

_____

_____

_____

_____

_____

Women's Beginner Routine · Phase 1 · Week 16

WORKOUT 1: LOWER BODY A

EXERCISES	SETS TOTAL WEIGHT X REPS, E.G., 45 X 12		
	SET 1	SET 2	SET 3
BODYWEIGHT LUNGE (WALKING) Warm-up and 3 hard sets of 12–15 reps	X	X	X
DUMBBELL DEADLIFT 3 hard sets of 12–15 reps	X	X	X
BODYWEIGHT SQUAT 3 hard sets of 12–15 reps	X	X	X
TRICEPS DIP 3 hard sets of 12–15 reps	X	X	X

NOTES

WORKOUT 2: UPPER BODY A

EXERCISES	SETS TOTAL WEIGHT X REPS, E.G., 45 X 12		
	SET 1	SET 2	SET 3
PUSH-UP Warm-up and 3 hard sets of 12–15 reps	X	X	X
ONE-ARM DUMBBELL ROW 3 hard sets of 12–15 reps	X	X	X

EXERCISES	SET 1	SET 2	SET 3
MACHINE SHOULDER PRESS 3 hard sets of 12–15 reps	X	X	X
BODYWEIGHT ROW 3 hard sets of 12–15 reps	X	X	X

NOTES

_____

_____

_____

_____

_____

WORKOUT 3: LOWER BODY B			
EXERCISES	**SETS** _TOTAL WEIGHT X REPS, E.G., 45 X 12_		
	SET 1	SET 2	SET 3
DUMBBELL DEADLIFT Warm-up and 3 hard sets of 12–15 reps	X	X	X
BODYWEIGHT STEP-UP 3 hard sets of 12–15 reps	X	X	X
LEG EXTENSION 3 hard sets of 12–15 reps	X	X	X
GLUTE BRIDGE 3 hard sets of 12–15 reps	X	X	X

NOTES

_____

_____

_____

_____

_____

Women's Beginner Routine · Phase 1 · Deload (Week 17)

WORKOUT 1: LOWER BODY A

EXERCISES	SETS *TOTAL WEIGHT X REPS, E.G., 45 X 12*	
	SET 1	SET 2
BODYWEIGHT LUNGE (WALKING) Warm-up and 2 hard sets of 10 reps	X	X
DUMBBELL DEADLIFT 2 hard sets of 10 reps	X	X
BODYWEIGHT SQUAT 2 hard sets of 10 reps	X	X
TRICEPS DIP 2 hard sets of 10 reps	X	X

NOTES

_____

_____

_____

_____

_____

_____

WORKOUT 2: UPPER BODY A

EXERCISES	SETS *TOTAL WEIGHT X REPS, E.G., 45 X 12*	
	SET 1	SET 2
PUSH-UP Warm-up and 2 hard sets of 10 reps	X	X
ONE-ARM DUMBBELL ROW 2 hard sets of 10 reps	X	X

EXERCISES	SET 1	SET 2
MACHINE SHOULDER PRESS 2 hard sets of 10 reps	X	X
BODYWEIGHT ROW 2 hard sets of 10 reps	X	X

NOTES

_____

_____

_____

_____

_____

WORKOUT 3: LOWER BODY B

EXERCISES	SETS *TOTAL WEIGHT X REPS, E.G., 45 X 12*	
	SET 1	SET 2
DUMBBELL DEADLIFT Warm-up and 2 hard sets of 10 reps	X	X
BODYWEIGHT STEP-UP 2 hard sets of 10 reps	X	X
LEG EXTENSION 2 hard sets of 10 reps	X	X
GLUTE BRIDGE 2 hard sets of 10 reps	X	X

NOTES

_____

_____

_____

_____

_____

FOUR MONTHS OF MEN'S BEGINNER WORKOUTS

Men's Beginner Routine · Phase 1 · Week 1

WORKOUT 1: UPPER BODY A

EXERCISES	SETS *TOTAL WEIGHT X REPS, E.G., 45 X 12*		
	SET 1	SET 2	SET 3
PUSH-UP Warm-up and 3 hard sets of 12–15 reps	X	X	X
LAT PULLDOWN 3 hard sets of 12–15 reps	X	X	X
MACHINE CHEST PRESS 3 hard sets of 12–15 reps	X	X	X
BODYWEIGHT ROW 3 hard sets of 12–15 reps	X	X	X

NOTES

_____

_____

_____

_____

_____

WORKOUT 2: LOWER BODY A

EXERCISES	SETS *TOTAL WEIGHT X REPS, E.G., 45 X 12*		
	SET 1	SET 2	SET 3
BODYWEIGHT SQUAT Warm-up and 3 hard sets of 12–15 reps	X	X	X
DUMBBELL DEADLIFT 3 hard sets of 12–15 reps	X	X	X

EXERCISES	SET 1	SET 2	SET 3
LEG PRESS 3 hard sets of 12–15 reps	X	X	X
LEG CURL (LYING OR SEATED) 3 hard sets of 12–15 reps	X	X	X

NOTES

_____

_____

_____

_____

_____

WORKOUT 3: UPPER BODY B			
EXERCISES	**SETS** _TOTAL WEIGHT X REPS, E.G., 45 X 12_		
	SET 1	SET 2	SET 3
MACHINE SHOULDER PRESS Warm-up and 3 hard sets of 12–15 reps	X	X	X
BODYWEIGHT ROW 3 hard sets of 12–15 reps	X	X	X
MACHINE CHEST PRESS 3 hard sets of 12–15 reps	X	X	X
CABLE BICEPS CURL 3 hard sets of 12–15 reps	X	X	X

NOTES

_____

_____

_____

_____

_____

Men's Beginner Routine · Phase 1 · Week 2

WORKOUT 1: UPPER BODY A			
EXERCISES	**SETS** *TOTAL WEIGHT X REPS, E.G., 45 X 12*		
	SET 1	**SET 2**	**SET 3**
PUSH-UP Warm-up and 3 hard sets of 12–15 reps	X	X	X
LAT PULLDOWN 3 hard sets of 12–15 reps	X	X	X
MACHINE CHEST PRESS 3 hard sets of 12–15 reps	X	X	X
BODYWEIGHT ROW 3 hard sets of 12–15 reps	X	X	X

NOTES

_____

_____

_____

_____

_____

_____

_____

WORKOUT 2: LOWER BODY A			
EXERCISES	**SETS** *TOTAL WEIGHT X REPS, E.G., 45 X 12*		
	SET 1	**SET 2**	**SET 3**
BODYWEIGHT SQUAT Warm-up and 3 hard sets of 12–15 reps	X	X	X
DUMBBELL DEADLIFT 3 hard sets of 12–15 reps	X	X	X

EXERCISES	SET 1	SET 2	SET 3
LEG PRESS 3 hard sets of 12–15 reps	X	X	X
LEG CURL (LYING OR SEATED) 3 hard sets of 12–15 reps	X	X	X

NOTES

_____

_____

_____

_____

_____

WORKOUT 3: UPPER BODY B

EXERCISES	SETS *TOTAL WEIGHT X REPS, E.G., 45 X 12*		
	SET 1	SET 2	SET 3
MACHINE SHOULDER PRESS Warm-up and 3 hard sets of 12–15 reps	X	X	X
BODYWEIGHT ROW 3 hard sets of 12–15 reps	X	X	X
MACHINE CHEST PRESS 3 hard sets of 12–15 reps	X	X	X
CABLE BICEPS CURL 3 hard sets of 12–15 reps	X	X	X

NOTES

_____

_____

_____

_____

_____

Men's Beginner Routine · Phase 1 · Week 3

WORKOUT 1: UPPER BODY A			
EXERCISES	**SETS** *TOTAL WEIGHT X REPS, E.G., 45 X 12*		
	SET 1	SET 2	SET 3
PUSH-UP Warm-up and 3 hard sets of 12–15 reps	X	X	X
LAT PULLDOWN 3 hard sets of 12–15 reps	X	X	X
MACHINE CHEST PRESS 3 hard sets of 12–15 reps	X	X	X
BODYWEIGHT ROW 3 hard sets of 12–15 reps	X	X	X

NOTES

_____

_____

_____

_____

_____

_____

_____

WORKOUT 2: LOWER BODY A			
EXERCISES	**SETS** *TOTAL WEIGHT X REPS, E.G., 45 X 12*		
	SET 1	SET 2	SET 3
BODYWEIGHT SQUAT Warm-up and 3 hard sets of 12–15 reps	X	X	X
DUMBBELL DEADLIFT 3 hard sets of 12–15 reps	X	X	X

EXERCISES	SET 1	SET 2	SET 3
LEG PRESS 3 hard sets of 12–15 reps	X	X	X
LEG CURL (LYING OR SEATED) 3 hard sets of 12–15 reps	X	X	X

NOTES

WORKOUT 3: UPPER BODY B			
EXERCISES	**SETS** *TOTAL WEIGHT X REPS, E.G., 45 X 12*		
	SET 1	SET 2	SET 3
MACHINE SHOULDER PRESS Warm-up and 3 hard sets of 12–15 reps	X	X	X
BODYWEIGHT ROW 3 hard sets of 12–15 reps	X	X	X
MACHINE CHEST PRESS 3 hard sets of 12–15 reps	X	X	X
CABLE BICEPS CURL 3 hard sets of 12–15 reps	X	X	X

NOTES

Men's Beginner Routine · Phase 1 · Week 4

WORKOUT 1: UPPER BODY A			
EXERCISES	**SETS** *TOTAL WEIGHT X REPS, E.G., 45 X 12*		
	SET 1	**SET 2**	**SET 3**
PUSH-UP Warm-up and 3 hard sets of 12–15 reps	X	X	X
LAT PULLDOWN 3 hard sets of 12–15 reps	X	X	X
MACHINE CHEST PRESS 3 hard sets of 12–15 reps	X	X	X
BODYWEIGHT ROW 3 hard sets of 12–15 reps	X	X	X

NOTES

_____

_____

_____

_____

_____

_____

WORKOUT 2: LOWER BODY A			
EXERCISES	**SETS** *TOTAL WEIGHT X REPS, E.G., 45 X 12*		
	SET 1	**SET 2**	**SET 3**
BODYWEIGHT SQUAT Warm-up and 3 hard sets of 12–15 reps	X	X	X
DUMBBELL DEADLIFT 3 hard sets of 12–15 reps	X	X	X

EXERCISES	SET 1	SET 2	SET 3
LEG PRESS 3 hard sets of 12–15 reps	X	X	X
LEG CURL (LYING OR SEATED) 3 hard sets of 12–15 reps	X	X	X

NOTES

_____

_____

_____

_____

WORKOUT 3: UPPER BODY B			
EXERCISES	**SETS** _TOTAL WEIGHT X REPS, E.G., 45 X 12_		
	SET 1	**SET 2**	**SET 3**
MACHINE SHOULDER PRESS Warm-up and 3 hard sets of 12–15 reps	X	X	X
BODYWEIGHT ROW 3 hard sets of 12–15 reps	X	X	X
MACHINE CHEST PRESS 3 hard sets of 12–15 reps	X	X	X
CABLE BICEPS CURL 3 hard sets of 12–15 reps	X	X	X

NOTES

_____

_____

_____

_____

_____

Men's Beginner Routine · Phase 1 · Week 5

WORKOUT 1: UPPER BODY A

EXERCISES	SETS TOTAL WEIGHT X REPS, E.G., 45 X 12		
	SET 1	SET 2	SET 3
PUSH-UP Warm-up and 3 hard sets of 12–15 reps	X	X	X
LAT PULLDOWN 3 hard sets of 12–15 reps	X	X	X
MACHINE CHEST PRESS 3 hard sets of 12–15 reps	X	X	X
BODYWEIGHT ROW 3 hard sets of 12–15 reps	X	X	X

NOTES

_____

_____

_____

_____

_____

_____

WORKOUT 2: LOWER BODY A

EXERCISES	SETS TOTAL WEIGHT X REPS, E.G., 45 X 12		
	SET 1	SET 2	SET 3
BODYWEIGHT SQUAT Warm-up and 3 hard sets of 12–15 reps	X	X	X
DUMBBELL DEADLIFT 3 hard sets of 12–15 reps	X	X	X

EXERCISES	SET 1	SET 2	SET 3
LEG PRESS 3 hard sets of 12–15 reps	X	X	X
LEG CURL (LYING OR SEATED) 3 hard sets of 12–15 reps	X	X	X

NOTES

_____

_____

_____

_____

_____

WORKOUT 3: UPPER BODY B

EXERCISES	SETS *TOTAL WEIGHT X REPS, E.G., 45 X 12*		
	SET 1	SET 2	SET 3
MACHINE SHOULDER PRESS Warm-up and 3 hard sets of 12–15 reps	X	X	X
BODYWEIGHT ROW 3 hard sets of 12–15 reps	X	X	X
MACHINE CHEST PRESS 3 hard sets of 12–15 reps	X	X	X
CABLE BICEPS CURL 3 hard sets of 12–15 reps	X	X	X

NOTES

_____

_____

_____

_____

_____

Men's Beginner Routine · Phase 1 · Week 6

WORKOUT 1: UPPER BODY A			
EXERCISES	**SETS** *TOTAL WEIGHT X REPS, E.G., 45 X 12*		
	SET 1	**SET 2**	**SET 3**
PUSH-UP Warm-up and 3 hard sets of 12–15 reps	X	X	X
LAT PULLDOWN 3 hard sets of 12–15 reps	X	X	X
MACHINE CHEST PRESS 3 hard sets of 12–15 reps	X	X	X
BODYWEIGHT ROW 3 hard sets of 12–15 reps	X	X	X

NOTES

_____

_____

_____

_____

_____

_____

_____

WORKOUT 2: LOWER BODY A			
EXERCISES	**SETS** *TOTAL WEIGHT X REPS, E.G., 45 X 12*		
	SET 1	**SET 2**	**SET 3**
BODYWEIGHT SQUAT Warm-up and 3 hard sets of 12–15 reps	X	X	X
DUMBBELL DEADLIFT 3 hard sets of 12–15 reps	X	X	X

EXERCISES	SET 1	SET 2	SET 3
LEG PRESS 3 hard sets of 12–15 reps	X	X	X
LEG CURL (LYING OR SEATED) 3 hard sets of 12–15 reps	X	X	X

NOTES

_____

_____

_____

_____

WORKOUT 3: UPPER BODY B			
EXERCISES	**SETS** _TOTAL WEIGHT X REPS, E.G., 45 X 12_		
	SET 1	**SET 2**	**SET 3**
MACHINE SHOULDER PRESS Warm-up and 3 hard sets of 12–15 reps	X	X	X
BODYWEIGHT ROW 3 hard sets of 12–15 reps	X	X	X
MACHINE CHEST PRESS 3 hard sets of 12–15 reps	X	X	X
CABLE BICEPS CURL 3 hard sets of 12–15 reps	X	X	X

NOTES

_____

_____

_____

_____

Men's Beginner Routine · Phase 1 · Week 7

WORKOUT 1: UPPER BODY A

EXERCISES	SETS TOTAL WEIGHT X REPS, E.G., 45 X 12		
	SET 1	SET 2	SET 3
PUSH-UP Warm-up and 3 hard sets of 12–15 reps	X	X	X
LAT PULLDOWN 3 hard sets of 12–15 reps	X	X	X
MACHINE CHEST PRESS 3 hard sets of 12–15 reps	X	X	X
BODYWEIGHT ROW 3 hard sets of 12–15 reps	X	X	X

NOTES

_____

_____

_____

_____

_____

_____

_____

WORKOUT 2: LOWER BODY A

EXERCISES	SETS TOTAL WEIGHT X REPS, E.G., 45 X 12		
	SET 1	SET 2	SET 3
BODYWEIGHT SQUAT Warm-up and 3 hard sets of 12–15 reps	X	X	X
DUMBBELL DEADLIFT 3 hard sets of 12–15 reps	X	X	X

EXERCISES	SET 1	SET 2	SET 3
LEG PRESS 3 hard sets of 12–15 reps	X	X	X
LEG CURL (LYING OR SEATED) 3 hard sets of 12–15 reps	X	X	X

NOTES

_____

_____

_____

_____

_____

WORKOUT 3: UPPER BODY B

EXERCISES	SETS *TOTAL WEIGHT X REPS, E.G., 45 X 12*		
	SET 1	SET 2	SET 3
MACHINE SHOULDER PRESS Warm-up and 3 hard sets of 12–15 reps	X	X	X
BODYWEIGHT ROW 3 hard sets of 12–15 reps	X	X	X
MACHINE CHEST PRESS 3 hard sets of 12–15 reps	X	X	X
CABLE BICEPS CURL 3 hard sets of 12–15 reps	X	X	X

NOTES

_____

_____

_____

_____

_____

Men's Beginner Routine · Phase 1 · Week 8

WORKOUT 1: UPPER BODY A

EXERCISES	SETS TOTAL WEIGHT X REPS, E.G., 45 X 12		
	SET 1	SET 2	SET 3
PUSH-UP Warm-up and 3 hard sets of 12–15 reps	X	X	X
LAT PULLDOWN 3 hard sets of 12–15 reps	X	X	X
MACHINE CHEST PRESS 3 hard sets of 12–15 reps	X	X	X
BODYWEIGHT ROW 3 hard sets of 12–15 reps	X	X	X

NOTES

_____

_____

_____

_____

_____

_____

WORKOUT 2: LOWER BODY A

EXERCISES	SETS TOTAL WEIGHT X REPS, E.G., 45 X 12		
	SET 1	SET 2	SET 3
BODYWEIGHT SQUAT Warm-up and 3 hard sets of 12–15 reps	X	X	X
DUMBBELL DEADLIFT 3 hard sets of 12–15 reps	X	X	X

MICHAEL MATTHEWS

EXERCISES	SET 1	SET 2	SET 3
LEG PRESS 3 hard sets of 12–15 reps	X	X	X
LEG CURL (LYING OR SEATED) 3 hard sets of 12–15 reps	X	X	X

NOTES

_____

_____

_____

_____

_____

WORKOUT 3: UPPER BODY B

EXERCISES	SETS _TOTAL WEIGHT X REPS, E.G., 45 X 12_		
	SET 1	SET 2	SET 3
MACHINE SHOULDER PRESS Warm-up and 3 hard sets of 12–15 reps	X	X	X
BODYWEIGHT ROW 3 hard sets of 12–15 reps	X	X	X
MACHINE CHEST PRESS 3 hard sets of 12–15 reps	X	X	X
CABLE BICEPS CURL 3 hard sets of 12–15 reps	X	X	X

NOTES

_____

_____

_____

_____

_____

Men's Beginner Routine · Phase 1 · Week 9

WORKOUT 1: UPPER BODY A			
EXERCISES	**SETS** *TOTAL WEIGHT X REPS, E.G., 45 X 12*		
	SET 1	**SET 2**	**SET 3**
PUSH-UP Warm-up and 3 hard sets of 12–15 reps	X	X	X
LAT PULLDOWN 3 hard sets of 12–15 reps	X	X	X
MACHINE SHOULDER PRESS 3 hard sets of 12–15 reps	X	X	X
ONE-ARM DUMBBELL ROW 3 hard sets of 12–15 reps	X	X	X

NOTES

_____

_____

_____

_____

_____

_____

WORKOUT 2: LOWER BODY A			
EXERCISES	**SETS** *TOTAL WEIGHT X REPS, E.G., 45 X 12*		
	SET 1	**SET 2**	**SET 3**
BODYWEIGHT SPLIT SQUAT Warm-up and 3 hard sets of 12–15 reps	X	X	X
DUMBBELL DEADLIFT 3 hard sets of 12–15 reps	X	X	X

EXERCISES	SET 1	SET 2	SET 3
LEG EXTENSION 3 hard sets of 12–15 reps	X	X	X
GLUTE BRIDGE 3 hard sets of 12–15 reps	X	X	X

NOTES

_____
_____
_____
_____
_____

WORKOUT 3: UPPER BODY B

EXERCISES	SETS *TOTAL WEIGHT X REPS, E.G., 45 X 12*		
	SET 1	SET 2	SET 3
MACHINE CHEST PRESS Warm-up and 3 hard sets of 12–15 reps	X	X	X
MACHINE ROW 3 hard sets of 12–15 reps	X	X	X
PUSH-UP 3 hard sets of 12–15 reps	X	X	X
ALTERNATING DUMBBELL CURL 3 hard sets of 12–15 reps	X	X	X

NOTES

_____
_____
_____
_____
_____

Men's Beginner Routine · Phase 1 · Week 10

WORKOUT 1: UPPER BODY A			
EXERCISES	**SETS** *TOTAL WEIGHT X REPS, E.G., 45 X 12*		
	SET 1	SET 2	SET 3
PUSH-UP Warm-up and 3 hard sets of 12–15 reps	X	X	X
LAT PULLDOWN 3 hard sets of 12–15 reps	X	X	X
MACHINE SHOULDER PRESS 3 hard sets of 12–15 reps	X	X	X
ONE-ARM DUMBBELL ROW 3 hard sets of 12–15 reps	X	X	X

NOTES

WORKOUT 2: LOWER BODY A			
EXERCISES	**SETS** *TOTAL WEIGHT X REPS, E.G., 45 X 12*		
	SET 1	SET 2	SET 3
BODYWEIGHT SPLIT SQUAT Warm-up and 3 hard sets of 12–15 reps	X	X	X
DUMBBELL DEADLIFT 3 hard sets of 12–15 reps	X	X	X

MICHAEL MATTHEWS

EXERCISES	SET 1	SET 2	SET 3
LEG EXTENSION 3 hard sets of 12–15 reps	X	X	X
GLUTE BRIDGE 3 hard sets of 12–15 reps	X	X	X

NOTES

WORKOUT 3: UPPER BODY B

EXERCISES	SETS *TOTAL WEIGHT X REPS, E.G., 45 X 12*		
	SET 1	SET 2	SET 3
MACHINE CHEST PRESS Warm-up and 3 hard sets of 12–15 reps	X	X	X
MACHINE ROW 3 hard sets of 12–15 reps	X	X	X
PUSH-UP 3 hard sets of 12–15 reps	X	X	X
ALTERNATING DUMBBELL CURL 3 hard sets of 12–15 reps	X	X	X

NOTES

Men's Beginner Routine · Phase 1 · Week 11

WORKOUT 1: UPPER BODY A

EXERCISES	SETS TOTAL WEIGHT X REPS, E.G., 45 X 12		
	SET 1	SET 2	SET 3
PUSH-UP Warm-up and 3 hard sets of 12–15 reps	X	X	X
LAT PULLDOWN 3 hard sets of 12–15 reps	X	X	X
MACHINE SHOULDER PRESS 3 hard sets of 12–15 reps	X	X	X
ONE-ARM DUMBBELL ROW 3 hard sets of 12–15 reps	X	X	X

NOTES

_____

_____

_____

_____

_____

_____

_____

WORKOUT 2: LOWER BODY A

EXERCISES	SETS TOTAL WEIGHT X REPS, E.G., 45 X 12		
	SET 1	SET 2	SET 3
BODYWEIGHT SPLIT SQUAT Warm-up and 3 hard sets of 12–15 reps	X	X	X
DUMBBELL DEADLIFT 3 hard sets of 12–15 reps	X	X	X

MICHAEL MATTHEWS

EXERCISES	SET 1	SET 2	SET 3
LEG EXTENSION 3 hard sets of 12–15 reps	X	X	X
GLUTE BRIDGE 3 hard sets of 12–15 reps	X	X	X

NOTES

_____

_____

_____

_____

_____

WORKOUT 3: UPPER BODY B

EXERCISES	SETS _TOTAL WEIGHT X REPS, E.G., 45 X 12_		
	SET 1	SET 2	SET 3
MACHINE CHEST PRESS Warm-up and 3 hard sets of 12–15 reps	X	X	X
MACHINE ROW 3 hard sets of 12–15 reps	X	X	X
PUSH-UP 3 hard sets of 12–15 reps	X	X	X
ALTERNATING DUMBBELL CURL 3 hard sets of 12–15 reps	X	X	X

NOTES

_____

_____

_____

_____

_____

Men's Beginner Routine · Phase 1 · Week 12

WORKOUT 1: UPPER BODY A			
EXERCISES	**SETS** *TOTAL WEIGHT X REPS, E.G., 45 X 12*		
	SET 1	**SET 2**	**SET 3**
PUSH-UP Warm-up and 3 hard sets of 12–15 reps	X	X	X
LAT PULLDOWN 3 hard sets of 12–15 reps	X	X	X
MACHINE SHOULDER PRESS 3 hard sets of 12–15 reps	X	X	X
ONE-ARM DUMBBELL ROW 3 hard sets of 12–15 reps	X	X	X

NOTES

WORKOUT 2: LOWER BODY A			
EXERCISES	**SETS** *TOTAL WEIGHT X REPS, E.G., 45 X 12*		
	SET 1	**SET 2**	**SET 3**
BODYWEIGHT SPLIT SQUAT Warm-up and 3 hard sets of 12–15 reps	X	X	X
DUMBBELL DEADLIFT 3 hard sets of 12–15 reps	X	X	X

EXERCISES	SET 1	SET 2	SET 3
LEG EXTENSION 3 hard sets of 12–15 reps	X	X	X
GLUTE BRIDGE 3 hard sets of 12–15 reps	X	X	X

NOTES

_____

_____

_____

_____

_____

WORKOUT 3: UPPER BODY B			
EXERCISES	**SETS** _TOTAL WEIGHT X REPS, E.G., 45 X 12_		
	SET 1	SET 2	SET 3
MACHINE CHEST PRESS Warm-up and 3 hard sets of 12–15 reps	X	X	X
MACHINE ROW 3 hard sets of 12–15 reps	X	X	X
PUSH-UP 3 hard sets of 12–15 reps	X	X	X
ALTERNATING DUMBBELL CURL 3 hard sets of 12–15 reps	X	X	X

NOTES

_____

_____

_____

_____

Men's Beginner Routine · Phase 1 · Week 13

WORKOUT 1: UPPER BODY A			
EXERCISES	**SETS** *TOTAL WEIGHT X REPS, E.G., 45 X 12*		
	SET 1	**SET 2**	**SET 3**
PUSH-UP Warm-up and 3 hard sets of 12–15 reps	X	X	X
LAT PULLDOWN 3 hard sets of 12–15 reps	X	X	X
MACHINE SHOULDER PRESS 3 hard sets of 12–15 reps	X	X	X
ONE-ARM DUMBBELL ROW 3 hard sets of 12–15 reps	X	X	X

NOTES

_____

_____

_____

_____

_____

_____

WORKOUT 2: LOWER BODY A			
EXERCISES	**SETS** *TOTAL WEIGHT X REPS, E.G., 45 X 12*		
	SET 1	**SET 2**	**SET 3**
BODYWEIGHT SPLIT SQUAT Warm-up and 3 hard sets of 12–15 reps	X	X	X
DUMBBELL DEADLIFT 3 hard sets of 12–15 reps	X	X	X

EXERCISES	SET 1	SET 2	SET 3
LEG EXTENSION 3 hard sets of 12–15 reps	X	X	X
GLUTE BRIDGE 3 hard sets of 12–15 reps	X	X	X

NOTES

_____

_____

_____

_____

_____

WORKOUT 3: UPPER BODY B			
EXERCISES	**SETS** _TOTAL WEIGHT X REPS, E.G., 45 X 12_		
	SET 1	SET 2	SET 3
MACHINE CHEST PRESS Warm-up and 3 hard sets of 12–15 reps	X	X	X
MACHINE ROW 3 hard sets of 12–15 reps	X	X	X
PUSH-UP 3 hard sets of 12–15 reps	X	X	X
ALTERNATING DUMBBELL CURL 3 hard sets of 12–15 reps	X	X	X

NOTES

_____

_____

_____

_____

_____

Men's Beginner Routine · Phase 1 · Week 14

WORKOUT 1: UPPER BODY A			
EXERCISES	**SETS** *TOTAL WEIGHT X REPS, E.G., 45 X 12*		
	SET 1	SET 2	SET 3
PUSH-UP Warm-up and 3 hard sets of 12–15 reps	X	X	X
LAT PULLDOWN 3 hard sets of 12–15 reps	X	X	X
MACHINE SHOULDER PRESS 3 hard sets of 12–15 reps	X	X	X
ONE-ARM DUMBBELL ROW 3 hard sets of 12–15 reps	X	X	X·

NOTES

_____

_____

_____

_____

_____

_____

WORKOUT 2: LOWER BODY A			
EXERCISES	**SETS** *TOTAL WEIGHT X REPS, E.G., 45 X 12*		
	SET 1	SET 2	SET 3
BODYWEIGHT SPLIT SQUAT Warm-up and 3 hard sets of 12–15 reps	X	X	X
DUMBBELL DEADLIFT 3 hard sets of 12–15 reps	X	X	X

EXERCISES	SET 1	SET 2	SET 3
LEG EXTENSION 3 hard sets of 12–15 reps	X	X	X
GLUTE BRIDGE 3 hard sets of 12–15 reps	X	X	X

NOTES

_____

_____

_____

_____

_____

WORKOUT 3: UPPER BODY B			
EXERCISES	**SETS** *TOTAL WEIGHT X REPS, E.G., 45 X 12*		
	SET 1	SET 2	SET 3
MACHINE CHEST PRESS Warm-up and 3 hard sets of 12–15 reps	X	X	X
MACHINE ROW 3 hard sets of 12–15 reps	X	X	X
PUSH-UP 3 hard sets of 12–15 reps	X	X	X
ALTERNATING DUMBBELL CURL 3 hard sets of 12–15 reps	X	X	X

NOTES

_____

_____

_____

_____

_____

Men's Beginner Routine · Phase 1 · Week 15

WORKOUT 1: UPPER BODY A			
EXERCISES	**SETS** *TOTAL WEIGHT X REPS, E.G., 45 X 12*		
	SET 1	**SET 2**	**SET 3**
PUSH-UP Warm-up and 3 hard sets of 12–15 reps	X	X	X
LAT PULLDOWN 3 hard sets of 12–15 reps	X	X	X
MACHINE SHOULDER PRESS 3 hard sets of 12–15 reps	X	X	X
ONE-ARM DUMBBELL ROW 3 hard sets of 12–15 reps	X	X	X

NOTES

_____

_____

_____

_____

_____

_____

WORKOUT 2: LOWER BODY A			
EXERCISES	**SETS** *TOTAL WEIGHT X REPS, E.G., 45 X 12*		
	SET 1	**SET 2**	**SET 3**
BODYWEIGHT SPLIT SQUAT Warm-up and 3 hard sets of 12–15 reps	X	X	X
DUMBBELL DEADLIFT 3 hard sets of 12–15 reps	X	X	X

EXERCISES	SET 1	SET 2	SET 3
LEG EXTENSION 3 hard sets of 12–15 reps	X	X	X
GLUTE BRIDGE 3 hard sets of 12–15 reps	X	X	X

NOTES

WORKOUT 3: UPPER BODY B

EXERCISES	SETS *TOTAL WEIGHT X REPS, E.G., 45 X 12*		
	SET 1	SET 2	SET 3
MACHINE CHEST PRESS Warm-up and 3 hard sets of 12–15 reps	X	X	X
MACHINE ROW 3 hard sets of 12–15 reps	X	X	X
PUSH-UP 3 hard sets of 12–15 reps	X	X	X
ALTERNATING DUMBBELL CURL 3 hard sets of 12–15 reps	X	X	X

NOTES

Men's Beginner Routine · Phase 1 · Week 16

WORKOUT 1: UPPER BODY A

EXERCISES	SETS *TOTAL WEIGHT X REPS, E.G., 45 X 12*		
	SET 1	SET 2	SET 3
PUSH-UP Warm-up and 3 hard sets of 12–15 reps	X	X	X
LAT PULLDOWN 3 hard sets of 12–15 reps	X	X	X
MACHINE SHOULDER PRESS 3 hard sets of 12–15 reps	X	X	X
ONE-ARM DUMBBELL ROW 3 hard sets of 12–15 reps	X	X	X

NOTES

_____

_____

_____

_____

_____

_____

WORKOUT 2: LOWER BODY A

EXERCISES	SETS *TOTAL WEIGHT X REPS, E.G., 45 X 12*		
	SET 1	SET 2	SET 3
BODYWEIGHT SPLIT SQUAT Warm-up and 3 hard sets of 12–15 reps	X	X	X
DUMBBELL DEADLIFT 3 hard sets of 12–15 reps	X	X	X

EXERCISES	SET 1	SET 2	SET 3
LEG EXTENSION 3 hard sets of 12–15 reps	X	X	X
GLUTE BRIDGE 3 hard sets of 12–15 reps	X	X	X

NOTES

_____

_____

_____

_____

_____

WORKOUT 3: UPPER BODY B			
EXERCISES	**SETS** _TOTAL WEIGHT X REPS, E.G., 45 X 12_		
	SET 1	SET 2	SET 3
MACHINE CHEST PRESS Warm-up and 3 hard sets of 12–15 reps	X	X	X
MACHINE ROW 3 hard sets of 12–15 reps	X	X	X
PUSH-UP 3 hard sets of 12–15 reps	X	X	X
ALTERNATING DUMBBELL CURL 3 hard sets of 12–15 reps	X	X	X

NOTES

_____

_____

_____

_____

_____

Men's Beginner Routine · Phase 1 · Deload (Week 17)

WORKOUT 1: UPPER BODY A		
EXERCISES	**SETS** *TOTAL WEIGHT X REPS, E.G., 45 X 12*	
	SET 1	SET 2
PUSH-UP Warm-up and 2 hard sets of 10 reps	X	X
LAT PULLDOWN 2 hard sets of 10 reps	X	X
MACHINE SHOULDER PRESS 2 hard sets of 10 reps	X	X
ONE-ARM DUMBBELL ROW 2 hard sets of 10 reps	X	X

NOTES

_____

_____

_____

_____

_____

_____

WORKOUT 2: LOWER BODY A		
EXERCISES	**SETS** *TOTAL WEIGHT X REPS, E.G., 45 X 12*	
	SET 1	SET 2
BODYWEIGHT SPLIT SQUAT Warm-up and 2 hard sets of 10 reps	X	X
DUMBBELL DEADLIFT 2 hard sets of 10 reps	X	X

EXERCISES	SET 1	SET 2
LEG EXTENSION 2 hard sets of 10 reps	X	X
GLUTE BRIDGE 2 hard sets of 10 reps	X	X

NOTES

WORKOUT 3: UPPER BODY B

EXERCISES	SETS *TOTAL WEIGHT X REPS, E.G., 45 X 12*	
	SET 1	SET 2
MACHINE CHEST PRESS Warm-up and 2 hard sets of 10 reps	X	X
MACHINE ROW 2 hard sets of 10 reps	X	X
PUSH-UP 2 hard sets of 10 reps	X	X
ALTERNATING DUMBBELL CURL 2 hard sets of 10 reps	X	X

NOTES

CONGRATULATIONS! YOU'VE COMPLETED PHASE ONE!

Phase One is done! Look at you!

Let's take a moment to think over what you've accomplished so far. You're now comfortable with the key exercises of the program and the weights you can handle, and you're also seeing clear improvements in your body composition and how your clothes fit.

Fun, right? And this is only the beginning!

Before we start your next training phase, let's see if we can help you get even more from it than you did from the first phase. Take a few minutes to reflect on the following questions and write down your answers so you can easily refer back to them as needed.

1. What are three things that went particularly well in the last phase? How so?

_____

_____

_____

_____

_____

2. What's at least one thing you could have done better? How so?

_____

_____

_____

_____

_____

3. What's at least one thing you can do to make your next phase even better than the last? To help you answer this productively, consider the following points:

· Has your training required a commute that's challenging or unsustainable? If so, can it be shortened?

- Has your training schedule fit in well with your other obligations? If not, can it be modified?
- Have any of the exercises in your workouts caused a significant amount of difficulty or discomfort? If so, what exercises given in chapter 2 can you substitute for them in this next phase?
- Have you had access to all of the equipment needed to do your workouts properly? If not, can you get access to that equipment?

_____

_____

_____

_____

_____

_____

Also, if you haven't taken any measurements and pictures yet (as discussed in chapter 4), here's a gentle reminder to do this now so you can start documenting your transformation with "hard evidence" that you'll begin to thrill at as you continue on the program.

Take the following body measurements as described in the same chapter:

DATE	WEIGHT		WAIST	CHEST
	SHOULDERS	UPPER LEGS	ARMS	CALVES

Also, you don't *have* to take all of these measurements if you don't want to, but you should at least record your weight and waist measurement.

Now let's discuss your next four months of training. So long as you meet the Phase Two strength standards shared in chapter 3 (virtually guaranteed by now), continue to Phase Two of the program. If you don't meet those standards yet, however, simply repeat Phase One again, and you should by the end of your second round.

You can also repeat Phase One if you just really enjoyed it or don't have access to the extra equipment required for Phase Two, but if you want to get the most out of your next training block, advance to the next phase of the program.

Oh, and finally, if you haven't already, find me on social media and let me know how you're doing on the program! If you're going to post about it, be sure to include the #muscleforlife hashtag, too, so other people looking for inspiration can find you and follow along, or connect with me on social media.

YOU KNOW
YOU'RE
GETTING
GOOD AT
THIS FITNESS
STUFF WHEN
IT'S HARDER
TO TAKE A
REST DAY
THAN TO DO
ANOTHER
WORKOUT.

FOUR MONTHS OF WOMEN'S INTERMEDIATE WORKOUTS
Women's Intermediate Routine · Phase 2 · Week 1

WORKOUT 1: LOWER BODY A			
EXERCISES	**SETS** *TOTAL WEIGHT X REPS, E.G., 45 X 12*		
	SET 1	**SET 2**	**SET 3**
TRAP-BAR DEADLIFT Warm-up and 3 hard sets of 10–12 reps	X	X	X
DUMBBELL SPLIT SQUAT 3 hard sets of 10–12 reps	X	X	X
LEG CURL (LYING OR SEATED) 3 hard sets of 10–12 reps	X	X	X
DUMBBELL GOBLET SQUAT 3 hard sets of 10–12 reps	X	X	X

NOTES

_____

_____

_____

_____

_____

WORKOUT 2: UPPER BODY A			
EXERCISES	**SETS** *TOTAL WEIGHT X REPS, E.G., 45 X 12*		
	SET 1	**SET 2**	**SET 3**
DUMBBELL BENCH PRESS Warm-up and 3 hard sets of 10–12 reps	X	X	X
LAT PULLDOWN 3 hard sets of 10–12 reps	X	X	X

MICHAEL MATTHEWS

EXERCISES	SET 1	SET 2	SET 3
SEATED DUMBBELL OVERHEAD PRESS 3 hard sets of 10–12 reps	X	X	X
SEATED CABLE ROW 3 hard sets of 10–12 reps	X	X	X

NOTES

_____

_____

_____

_____

WORKOUT 3: LOWER BODY B

EXERCISES	SETS _TOTAL WEIGHT X REPS, E.G., 45 X 12_		
	SET 1	SET 2	SET 3
DUMBBELL LUNGE (IN-PLACE) Warm-up and 3 hard sets of 10–12 reps	X	X	X
DUMBBELL ROMANIAN DEADLIFT 3 hard sets of 10–12 reps	X	X	X
LEG PRESS 3 hard sets of 10–12 reps	X	X	X
LEG CURL (LYING OR SEATED) 3 hard sets of 10–12 reps	X	X	X

NOTES

_____

_____

_____

_____

_____

Women's Intermediate Routine · Phase 2 · Week 2

WORKOUT 1: LOWER BODY A

EXERCISES	SETS TOTAL WEIGHT X REPS, E.G., 45 X 12		
	SET 1	SET 2	SET 3
TRAP-BAR DEADLIFT Warm-up and 3 hard sets of 10–12 reps	X	X	X
DUMBBELL SPLIT SQUAT 3 hard sets of 10–12 reps	X	X	X
LEG CURL (LYING OR SEATED) 3 hard sets of 10–12 reps	X	X	X
DUMBBELL GOBLET SQUAT 3 hard sets of 10–12 reps	X	X	X

NOTES

_____

_____

_____

_____

_____

_____

_____

WORKOUT 2: UPPER BODY A

EXERCISES	SETS TOTAL WEIGHT X REPS, E.G., 45 X 12		
	SET 1	SET 2	SET 3
DUMBBELL BENCH PRESS Warm-up and 3 hard sets of 10–12 reps	X	X	X
LAT PULLDOWN 3 hard sets of 10–12 reps	X	X	X

EXERCISES	SET 1	SET 2	SET 3
SEATED DUMBBELL OVERHEAD PRESS 3 hard sets of 10–12 reps	X	X	X
SEATED CABLE ROW 3 hard sets of 10–12 reps	X	X	X

NOTES

_____
_____
_____
_____
_____

WORKOUT 3: LOWER BODY B			
EXERCISES	**SETS** _TOTAL WEIGHT X REPS, E.G., 45 X 12_		
	SET 1	SET 2	SET 3
DUMBBELL LUNGE (IN-PLACE) Warm-up and 3 hard sets of 10–12 reps	X	X	X
DUMBBELL ROMANIAN DEADLIFT 3 hard sets of 10–12 reps	X	X	X
LEG PRESS 3 hard sets of 10–12 reps	X	X	X
LEG CURL (LYING OR SEATED) 3 hard sets of 10–12 reps	X	X	X

NOTES

_____
_____
_____
_____
_____

Women's Intermediate Routine · Phase 2 · Week 3

WORKOUT 1: LOWER BODY A			
EXERCISES	**SETS** *TOTAL WEIGHT X REPS, E.G., 45 X 12*		
	SET 1	SET 2	SET 3
TRAP-BAR DEADLIFT Warm-up and 3 hard sets of 10–12 reps	X	X	X
DUMBBELL SPLIT SQUAT 3 hard sets of 10–12 reps	X	X	X
LEG CURL (LYING OR SEATED) 3 hard sets of 10–12 reps	X	X	X
DUMBBELL GOBLET SQUAT 3 hard sets of 10–12 reps	X	X	X

NOTES

_____

_____

_____

_____

_____

_____

WORKOUT 2: UPPER BODY A			
EXERCISES	**SETS** *TOTAL WEIGHT X REPS, E.G., 45 X 12*		
	SET 1	SET 2	SET 3
DUMBBELL BENCH PRESS Warm-up and 3 hard sets of 10–12 reps	X	X	X
LAT PULLDOWN 3 hard sets of 10–12 reps	X	X	X

EXERCISES	SET 1	SET 2	SET 3
SEATED DUMBBELL OVERHEAD PRESS 3 hard sets of 10–12 reps	X	X	X
SEATED CABLE ROW 3 hard sets of 10–12 reps	X	X	X

NOTES

_____

_____

_____

_____

_____

WORKOUT 3: LOWER BODY B

EXERCISES	SETS _TOTAL WEIGHT X REPS, E.G., 45 X 12_		
	SET 1	SET 2	SET 3
DUMBBELL LUNGE (IN-PLACE) Warm-up and 3 hard sets of 10–12 reps	X	X	X
DUMBBELL ROMANIAN DEADLIFT 3 hard sets of 10–12 reps	X	X	X
LEG PRESS 3 hard sets of 10–12 reps	X	X	X
LEG CURL (LYING OR SEATED) 3 hard sets of 10–12 reps	X	X	X

NOTES

_____

_____

_____

_____

_____

Women's Intermediate Routine · Phase 2 · Week 4

WORKOUT 1: LOWER BODY A			
EXERCISES	**SETS** *TOTAL WEIGHT X REPS, E.G., 45 X 12*		
	SET 1	**SET 2**	**SET 3**
TRAP-BAR DEADLIFT Warm-up and 3 hard sets of 10–12 reps	X	X	X
DUMBBELL SPLIT SQUAT 3 hard sets of 10–12 reps	X	X	X
LEG CURL (LYING OR SEATED) 3 hard sets of 10–12 reps	X	X	X
DUMBBELL GOBLET SQUAT 3 hard sets of 10–12 reps	X	X	X

NOTES

_____

_____

_____

_____

_____

_____

WORKOUT 2: UPPER BODY A			
EXERCISES	**SETS** *TOTAL WEIGHT X REPS, E.G., 45 X 12*		
	SET 1	**SET 2**	**SET 3**
DUMBBELL BENCH PRESS Warm-up and 3 hard sets of 10–12 reps	X	X	X
LAT PULLDOWN 3 hard sets of 10–12 reps	X	X	X

EXERCISES	SET 1	SET 2	SET 3
SEATED DUMBBELL OVERHEAD PRESS 3 hard sets of 10–12 reps	X	X	X
SEATED CABLE ROW 3 hard sets of 10–12 reps	X	X	X

NOTES

_____

_____

_____

_____

_____

WORKOUT 3: LOWER BODY B			
EXERCISES	**SETS** _TOTAL WEIGHT X REPS, E.G., 45 X 12_		
	SET 1	SET 2	SET 3
DUMBBELL LUNGE (IN-PLACE) Warm-up and 3 hard sets of 10–12 reps	X	X	X
DUMBBELL ROMANIAN DEADLIFT 3 hard sets of 10–12 reps	X	X	X
LEG PRESS 3 hard sets of 10–12 reps	X	X	X
LEG CURL (LYING OR SEATED) 3 hard sets of 10–12 reps	X	X	X

NOTES

_____

_____

_____

_____

_____

Women's Intermediate Routine · Phase 2 · Week 5

WORKOUT 1: LOWER BODY A			
EXERCISES	**SETS** *TOTAL WEIGHT X REPS, E.G., 45 X 12*		
	SET 1	**SET 2**	**SET 3**
TRAP-BAR DEADLIFT Warm-up and 3 hard sets of 10–12 reps	X	X	X
DUMBBELL SPLIT SQUAT 3 hard sets of 10–12 reps	X	X	X
LEG CURL (LYING OR SEATED) 3 hard sets of 10–12 reps	X	X	X
DUMBBELL GOBLET SQUAT 3 hard sets of 10–12 reps	X	X	X

NOTES

_____

_____

_____

_____

_____

_____

_____

WORKOUT 2: UPPER BODY A			
EXERCISES	**SETS** *TOTAL WEIGHT X REPS, E.G., 45 X 12*		
	SET 1	**SET 2**	**SET 3**
DUMBBELL BENCH PRESS Warm-up and 3 hard sets of 10–12 reps	X	X	X
LAT PULLDOWN 3 hard sets of 10–12 reps	X	X	X

EXERCISES	SET 1	SET 2	SET 3
SEATED DUMBBELL OVERHEAD PRESS 3 hard sets of 10–12 reps	X	X	X
SEATED CABLE ROW 3 hard sets of 10–12 reps	X	X	X

NOTES

WORKOUT 3: LOWER BODY B

EXERCISES	SETS *TOTAL WEIGHT X REPS, E.G., 45 X 12*		
	SET 1	SET 2	SET 3
DUMBBELL LUNGE (IN-PLACE) Warm-up and 3 hard sets of 10–12 reps	X	X	X
DUMBBELL ROMANIAN DEADLIFT 3 hard sets of 10–12 reps	X	X	X
LEG PRESS 3 hard sets of 10–12 reps	X	X	X
LEG CURL (LYING OR SEATED) 3 hard sets of 10–12 reps	X	X	X

NOTES

Women's Intermediate Routine · Phase 2 · Week 6

WORKOUT 1: LOWER BODY A			
EXERCISES	**SETS** *TOTAL WEIGHT X REPS, E.G., 45 X 12*		
	SET 1	SET 2	SET 3
TRAP-BAR DEADLIFT Warm-up and 3 hard sets of 10–12 reps	X	X	X
DUMBBELL SPLIT SQUAT 3 hard sets of 10–12 reps	X	X	X
LEG CURL (LYING OR SEATED) 3 hard sets of 10–12 reps	X	X	X
DUMBBELL GOBLET SQUAT 3 hard sets of 10–12 reps	X	X	X

NOTES

_____

_____

_____

_____

_____

_____

_____

WORKOUT 2: UPPER BODY A			
EXERCISES	**SETS** *TOTAL WEIGHT X REPS, E.G., 45 X 12*		
	SET 1	SET 2	SET 3
DUMBBELL BENCH PRESS Warm-up and 3 hard sets of 10–12 reps	X	X	X
LAT PULLDOWN 3 hard sets of 10–12 reps	X	X	X

EXERCISES	SET 1	SET 2	SET 3
SEATED DUMBBELL OVERHEAD PRESS 3 hard sets of 10–12 reps	X	X	X
SEATED CABLE ROW 3 hard sets of 10–12 reps	X	X	X

NOTES

_____

_____

_____

_____

_____

WORKOUT 3: LOWER BODY B

EXERCISES	SETS _TOTAL WEIGHT X REPS, E.G., 45 X 12_		
	SET 1	SET 2	SET 3
DUMBBELL LUNGE (IN-PLACE) Warm-up and 3 hard sets of 10–12 reps	X	X	X
DUMBBELL ROMANIAN DEADLIFT 3 hard sets of 10–12 reps	X	X	X
LEG PRESS 3 hard sets of 10–12 reps	X	X	X
LEG CURL (LYING OR SEATED) 3 hard sets of 10–12 reps	X	X	X

NOTES

_____

_____

_____

_____

_____

Women's Intermediate Routine · Phase 2 · Week 7

WORKOUT 1: LOWER BODY A			
EXERCISES	**SETS** *TOTAL WEIGHT X REPS, E.G., 45 X 12*		
	SET 1	SET 2	SET 3
TRAP-BAR DEADLIFT Warm-up and 3 hard sets of 10–12 reps	X	X	X
DUMBBELL SPLIT SQUAT 3 hard sets of 10–12 reps	X	X	X
LEG CURL (LYING OR SEATED) 3 hard sets of 10–12 reps	X	X	X
DUMBBELL GOBLET SQUAT 3 hard sets of 10–12 reps	X	X	X

NOTES

_____

_____

_____

_____

_____

_____

_____

WORKOUT 2: UPPER BODY A			
EXERCISES	**SETS** *TOTAL WEIGHT X REPS, E.G., 45 X 12*		
	SET 1	SET 2	SET 3
DUMBBELL BENCH PRESS Warm-up and 3 hard sets of 10–12 reps	X	X	X
LAT PULLDOWN 3 hard sets of 10–12 reps	X	X	X

EXERCISES	SET 1	SET 2	SET 3
SEATED DUMBBELL OVERHEAD PRESS 3 hard sets of 10–12 reps	X	X	X
SEATED CABLE ROW 3 hard sets of 10–12 reps	X	X	X

NOTES

_____

_____

_____

_____

_____

WORKOUT 3: LOWER BODY B

EXERCISES	SETS *TOTAL WEIGHT X REPS, E.G., 45 X 12*		
	SET 1	SET 2	SET 3
DUMBBELL LUNGE (IN-PLACE) Warm-up and 3 hard sets of 10–12 reps	X	X	X
DUMBBELL ROMANIAN DEADLIFT 3 hard sets of 10–12 reps	X	X	X
LEG PRESS 3 hard sets of 10–12 reps	X	X	X
LEG CURL (LYING OR SEATED) 3 hard sets of 10–12 reps	X	X	X

NOTES

_____

_____

_____

_____

_____

Women's Intermediate Routine · Phase 2 · Week 8

WORKOUT 1: LOWER BODY A			
EXERCISES	**SETS** *TOTAL WEIGHT X REPS, E.G., 45 X 12*		
	SET 1	**SET 2**	**SET 3**
TRAP-BAR DEADLIFT Warm-up and 3 hard sets of 10–12 reps	X	X	X
DUMBBELL SPLIT SQUAT 3 hard sets of 10–12 reps	X	X	X
LEG CURL (LYING OR SEATED) 3 hard sets of 10–12 reps	X	X	X
DUMBBELL GOBLET SQUAT 3 hard sets of 10–12 reps	X	X	X

NOTES

_____

_____

_____

_____

_____

_____

WORKOUT 2: UPPER BODY A			
EXERCISES	**SETS** *TOTAL WEIGHT X REPS, E.G., 45 X 12*		
	SET 1	**SET 2**	**SET 3**
DUMBBELL BENCH PRESS Warm-up and 3 hard sets of 10–12 reps	X	X	X
LAT PULLDOWN 3 hard sets of 10–12 reps	X	X	X

EXERCISES	SET 1	SET 2	SET 3
SEATED DUMBBELL OVERHEAD PRESS 3 hard sets of 10–12 reps	X	X	X
SEATED CABLE ROW 3 hard sets of 10–12 reps	X	X	X

NOTES

_____

_____

_____

_____

_____

WORKOUT 3: LOWER BODY B

EXERCISES	SETS *TOTAL WEIGHT X REPS, E.G., 45 X 12*		
	SET 1	SET 2	SET 3
DUMBBELL LUNGE (IN-PLACE) Warm-up and 3 hard sets of 10–12 reps	X	X	X
DUMBBELL ROMANIAN DEADLIFT 3 hard sets of 10–12 reps	X	X	X
LEG PRESS 3 hard sets of 10–12 reps	X	X	X
LEG CURL (LYING OR SEATED) 3 hard sets of 10–12 reps	X	X	X

NOTES

_____

_____

_____

_____

_____

Women's Intermediate Routine · Phase 2 · Week 9

WORKOUT 1: LOWER BODY A			
EXERCISES	**SETS** *TOTAL WEIGHT X REPS, E.G., 45 X 12*		
	SET 1	SET 2	SET 3
TRAP-BAR DEADLIFT Warm-up and 3 hard sets of 10–12 reps	X	X	X
DUMBBELL LUNGE (WALKING) 3 hard sets of 10–12 reps	X	X	X
DUMBBELL ROMANIAN DEADLIFT 3 hard sets of 10–12 reps	X	X	X
DUMBBELL GOBLET SQUAT 3 hard sets of 10–12 reps	X	X	X

NOTES

_____

_____

_____

_____

_____

_____

WORKOUT 2: UPPER BODY A			
EXERCISES	**SETS** *TOTAL WEIGHT X REPS, E.G., 45 X 12*		
	SET 1	SET 2	SET 3
INCLINE DUMBBELL BENCH PRESS Warm-up and 3 hard sets of 10–12 reps	X	X	X
ONE-ARM DUMBBELL ROW 3 hard sets of 10–12 reps	X	X	X

EXERCISES	SET 1	SET 2	SET 3
DUMBBELL BENCH PRESS 3 hard sets of 10–12 reps	X	X	X
SEATED CABLE ROW 3 hard sets of 10–12 reps	X	X	X

NOTES

_____

_____

_____

_____

_____

WORKOUT 3: LOWER BODY B			
EXERCISES	**SETS** _TOTAL WEIGHT X REPS, E.G., 45 X 12_		
	SET 1	SET 2	SET 3
DUMBBELL GOBLET SQUAT Warm-up and 3 hard sets of 10–12 reps	X	X	X
DUMBBELL DEADLIFT 3 hard sets of 10–12 reps	X	X	X
LEG EXTENSION 3 hard sets of 10–12 reps	X	X	X
LEG CURL (LYING OR SEATED) 3 hard sets of 10–12 reps	X	X	X

NOTES

_____

_____

_____

_____

_____

Women's Intermediate Routine · Phase 2 · Week 10

WORKOUT 1: LOWER BODY A			
EXERCISES	**SETS** *TOTAL WEIGHT X REPS, E.G., 45 X 12*		
	SET 1	SET 2	SET 3
TRAP-BAR DEADLIFT Warm-up and 3 hard sets of 10–12 reps	X	X	X
DUMBBELL LUNGE (WALKING) 3 hard sets of 10–12 reps	X	X	X
DUMBBELL ROMANIAN DEADLIFT 3 hard sets of 10–12 reps	X	X	X
DUMBBELL GOBLET SQUAT 3 hard sets of 10–12 reps	X	X	X

NOTES

WORKOUT 2: UPPER BODY A			
EXERCISES	**SETS** *TOTAL WEIGHT X REPS, E.G., 45 X 12*		
	SET 1	SET 2	SET 3
INCLINE DUMBBELL BENCH PRESS Warm-up and 3 hard sets of 10–12 reps	X	X	X
ONE-ARM DUMBBELL ROW 3 hard sets of 10–12 reps	X	X	X

EXERCISES	SET 1	SET 2	SET 3
DUMBBELL BENCH PRESS 3 hard sets of 10–12 reps	X	X	X
SEATED CABLE ROW 3 hard sets of 10–12 reps	X	X	X

NOTES

_____

_____

_____

_____

WORKOUT 3: LOWER BODY B

EXERCISES	SETS *TOTAL WEIGHT X REPS, E.G., 45 X 12*		
	SET 1	SET 2	SET 3
DUMBBELL GOBLET SQUAT Warm-up and 3 hard sets of 10–12 reps	X	X	X
DUMBBELL DEADLIFT 3 hard sets of 10–12 reps	X	X	X
LEG EXTENSION 3 hard sets of 10–12 reps	X	X	X
LEG CURL (LYING OR SEATED) 3 hard sets of 10–12 reps	X	X	X

NOTES

_____

_____

_____

_____

Women's Intermediate Routine · Phase 2 · Week 11

WORKOUT 1: LOWER BODY A			
EXERCISES	**SETS** _TOTAL WEIGHT X REPS, E.G., 45 X 12_		
	SET 1	**SET 2**	**SET 3**
TRAP-BAR DEADLIFT Warm-up and 3 hard sets of 10–12 reps	X	X	X
DUMBBELL LUNGE (WALKING) 3 hard sets of 10–12 reps	X	X	X
DUMBBELL ROMANIAN DEADLIFT 3 hard sets of 10–12 reps	X	X	X
DUMBBELL GOBLET SQUAT 3 hard sets of 10–12 reps	X	X	X

NOTES

_____

_____

_____

_____

_____

_____

WORKOUT 2: UPPER BODY A			
EXERCISES	**SETS** _TOTAL WEIGHT X REPS, E.G., 45 X 12_		
	SET 1	**SET 2**	**SET 3**
INCLINE DUMBBELL BENCH PRESS Warm-up and 3 hard sets of 10–12 reps	X	X	X
ONE-ARM DUMBBELL ROW 3 hard sets of 10–12 reps	X	X	X

EXERCISES	SET 1	SET 2	SET 3
DUMBBELL BENCH PRESS 3 hard sets of 10–12 reps	X	X	X
SEATED CABLE ROW 3 hard sets of 10–12 reps	X	X	X

NOTES

_____

_____

_____

_____

WORKOUT 3: LOWER BODY B			
EXERCISES	**SETS** *TOTAL WEIGHT X REPS, E.G., 45 X 12*		
	SET 1	SET 2	SET 3
DUMBBELL GOBLET SQUAT Warm-up and 3 hard sets of 10–12 reps	X	X	X
DUMBBELL DEADLIFT 3 hard sets of 10–12 reps	X	X	X
LEG EXTENSION 3 hard sets of 10–12 reps	X	X	X
LEG CURL (LYING OR SEATED) 3 hard sets of 10–12 reps	X	X	X

NOTES

_____

_____

_____

_____

Women's Intermediate Routine · Phase 2 · Week 12

WORKOUT 1: LOWER BODY A			
EXERCISES	**SETS** *TOTAL WEIGHT X REPS, E.G., 45 X 12*		
	SET 1	**SET 2**	**SET 3**
TRAP-BAR DEADLIFT Warm-up and 3 hard sets of 10–12 reps	X	X	X
DUMBBELL LUNGE (WALKING) 3 hard sets of 10–12 reps	X	X	X
DUMBBELL ROMANIAN DEADLIFT 3 hard sets of 10–12 reps	X	X	X
DUMBBELL GOBLET SQUAT 3 hard sets of 10–12 reps	X	X	X

NOTES

_____

_____

_____

_____

_____

_____

_____

WORKOUT 2: UPPER BODY A			
EXERCISES	**SETS** *TOTAL WEIGHT X REPS, E.G., 45 X 12*		
	SET 1	**SET 2**	**SET 3**
INCLINE DUMBBELL BENCH PRESS Warm-up and 3 hard sets of 10–12 reps	X	X	X
ONE-ARM DUMBBELL ROW 3 hard sets of 10–12 reps	X	X	X

EXERCISES	SET 1	SET 2	SET 3
DUMBBELL BENCH PRESS 3 hard sets of 10–12 reps	X	X	X
SEATED CABLE ROW 3 hard sets of 10–12 reps	X	X	X

NOTES

WORKOUT 3: LOWER BODY B			
EXERCISES	**SETS** *TOTAL WEIGHT X REPS, E.G., 45 X 12*		
	SET 1	SET 2	SET 3
DUMBBELL GOBLET SQUAT Warm-up and 3 hard sets of 10–12 reps	X	X	X
DUMBBELL DEADLIFT 3 hard sets of 10–12 reps	X	X	X
LEG EXTENSION 3 hard sets of 10–12 reps	X	X	X
LEG CURL (LYING OR SEATED) 3 hard sets of 10–12 reps	X	X	X

NOTES

Women's Intermediate Routine · Phase 2 · Week 13

WORKOUT 1: LOWER BODY A			
EXERCISES	**SETS** *TOTAL WEIGHT X REPS, E.G., 45 X 12*		
	SET 1	**SET 2**	**SET 3**
TRAP-BAR DEADLIFT Warm-up and 3 hard sets of 10–12 reps	X	X	X
DUMBBELL LUNGE (WALKING) 3 hard sets of 10–12 reps	X	X	X
DUMBBELL ROMANIAN DEADLIFT 3 hard sets of 10–12 reps	X	X	X
DUMBBELL GOBLET SQUAT 3 hard sets of 10–12 reps	X	X	X

NOTES

_____

_____

_____

_____

_____

_____

_____

WORKOUT 2: UPPER BODY A			
EXERCISES	**SETS** *TOTAL WEIGHT X REPS, E.G., 45 X 12*		
	SET 1	**SET 2**	**SET 3**
INCLINE DUMBBELL BENCH PRESS Warm-up and 3 hard sets of 10–12 reps	X	X	X
ONE-ARM DUMBBELL ROW 3 hard sets of 10–12 reps	X	X	X

EXERCISES	SET 1	SET 2	SET 3
DUMBBELL BENCH PRESS 3 hard sets of 10–12 reps	X	X	X
SEATED CABLE ROW 3 hard sets of 10–12 reps	X	X	X

NOTES

_____

_____

_____

_____

_____

WORKOUT 3: LOWER BODY B			
EXERCISES	**SETS** _TOTAL WEIGHT X REPS, E.G., 45 X 12_		
	SET 1	SET 2	SET 3
DUMBBELL GOBLET SQUAT Warm-up and 3 hard sets of 10–12 reps	X	X	X
DUMBBELL DEADLIFT 3 hard sets of 10–12 reps	X	X	X
LEG EXTENSION 3 hard sets of 10–12 reps	X	X	X
LEG CURL (LYING OR SEATED) 3 hard sets of 10–12 reps	X	X	X

NOTES

_____

_____

_____

_____

_____

Women's Intermediate Routine · Phase 2 · Week 14

WORKOUT 1: LOWER BODY A			
EXERCISES	**SETS** *TOTAL WEIGHT X REPS, E.G., 45 X 12*		
	SET 1	**SET 2**	**SET 3**
TRAP-BAR DEADLIFT Warm-up and 3 hard sets of 10–12 reps	X	X	X
DUMBBELL LUNGE (WALKING) 3 hard sets of 10–12 reps	X	X	X
DUMBBELL ROMANIAN DEADLIFT 3 hard sets of 10–12 reps	X	X	X
DUMBBELL GOBLET SQUAT 3 hard sets of 10–12 reps	X	X	X

NOTES

_____

_____

_____

_____

_____

_____

_____

WORKOUT 2: UPPER BODY A			
EXERCISES	**SETS** *TOTAL WEIGHT X REPS, E.G., 45 X 12*		
	SET 1	**SET 2**	**SET 3**
INCLINE DUMBBELL BENCH PRESS Warm-up and 3 hard sets of 10–12 reps	X	X	X
ONE-ARM DUMBBELL ROW 3 hard sets of 10–12 reps	X	X	X

MICHAEL MATTHEWS

EXERCISES	SET 1	SET 2	SET 3
DUMBBELL BENCH PRESS 3 hard sets of 10–12 reps	X	X	X
SEATED CABLE ROW 3 hard sets of 10–12 reps	X	X	X

NOTES

_____

_____

_____

_____

WORKOUT 3: LOWER BODY B			
EXERCISES	**SETS** _TOTAL WEIGHT X REPS, E.G., 45 X 12_		
	SET 1	SET 2	SET 3
DUMBBELL GOBLET SQUAT Warm-up and 3 hard sets of 10–12 reps	X	X	X
DUMBBELL DEADLIFT 3 hard sets of 10–12 reps	X	X	X
LEG EXTENSION 3 hard sets of 10–12 reps	X	X	X
LEG CURL (LYING OR SEATED) 3 hard sets of 10–12 reps	X	X	X

NOTES

_____

_____

_____

_____

_____

Women's Intermediate Routine · Phase 2 · Week 15

WORKOUT 1: LOWER BODY A			
EXERCISES	**SETS** *TOTAL WEIGHT X REPS, E.G., 45 X 12*		
	SET 1	**SET 2**	**SET 3**
TRAP-BAR DEADLIFT Warm-up and 3 hard sets of 10–12 reps	X	X	X
DUMBBELL LUNGE (WALKING) 3 hard sets of 10–12 reps	X	X	X
DUMBBELL ROMANIAN DEADLIFT 3 hard sets of 10–12 reps	X	X	X
DUMBBELL GOBLET SQUAT 3 hard sets of 10–12 reps	X	X	X

NOTES

_____

_____

_____

_____

_____

_____

WORKOUT 2: UPPER BODY A			
EXERCISES	**SETS** *TOTAL WEIGHT X REPS, E.G., 45 X 12*		
	SET 1	**SET 2**	**SET 3**
INCLINE DUMBBELL BENCH PRESS Warm-up and 3 hard sets of 10–12 reps	X	X	X
ONE-ARM DUMBBELL ROW 3 hard sets of 10–12 reps	X	X	X

EXERCISES	SET 1	SET 2	SET 3
DUMBBELL BENCH PRESS 3 hard sets of 10–12 reps	X	X	X
SEATED CABLE ROW 3 hard sets of 10–12 reps	X	X	X

NOTES

_____

_____

_____

_____

WORKOUT 3: LOWER BODY B			
EXERCISES	**SETS** _TOTAL WEIGHT X REPS, E.G., 45 X 12_		
	SET 1	SET 2	SET 3
DUMBBELL GOBLET SQUAT Warm-up and 3 hard sets of 10–12 reps	X	X	X
DUMBBELL DEADLIFT 3 hard sets of 10–12 reps	X	X	X
LEG EXTENSION 3 hard sets of 10–12 reps	X	X	X
LEG CURL (LYING OR SEATED) 3 hard sets of 10–12 reps	X	X	X

NOTES

_____

_____

_____

_____

_____

Women's Intermediate Routine · Phase 2 · Week 16

WORKOUT 1: LOWER BODY A			
EXERCISES	**SETS** *TOTAL WEIGHT X REPS, E.G., 45 X 12*		
	SET 1	SET 2	SET 3
TRAP-BAR DEADLIFT Warm-up and 3 hard sets of 10–12 reps	X	X	X
DUMBBELL LUNGE (WALKING) 3 hard sets of 10–12 reps	X	X	X
DUMBBELL ROMANIAN DEADLIFT 3 hard sets of 10–12 reps	X	X	X
DUMBBELL GOBLET SQUAT 3 hard sets of 10–12 reps	X	X	X

NOTES

_____

_____

_____

_____

_____

_____

_____

WORKOUT 2: UPPER BODY A			
EXERCISES	**SETS** *TOTAL WEIGHT X REPS, E.G., 45 X 12*		
	SET 1	SET 2	SET 3
INCLINE DUMBBELL BENCH PRESS Warm-up and 3 hard sets of 10–12 reps	X	X	X
ONE-ARM DUMBBELL ROW 3 hard sets of 10–12 reps	X	X	X

EXERCISES	SET 1	SET 2	SET 3
DUMBBELL BENCH PRESS 3 hard sets of 10–12 reps	X	X	X
SEATED CABLE ROW 3 hard sets of 10–12 reps	X	X	X

NOTES

_____

_____

_____

_____

_____

WORKOUT 3: LOWER BODY B			
EXERCISES	**SETS** *TOTAL WEIGHT X REPS, E.G., 45 X 12*		
	SET 1	SET 2	SET 3
DUMBBELL GOBLET SQUAT Warm-up and 3 hard sets of 10–12 reps	X	X	X
DUMBBELL DEADLIFT 3 hard sets of 10–12 reps	X	X	X
LEG EXTENSION 3 hard sets of 10–12 reps	X	X	X
LEG CURL (LYING OR SEATED) 3 hard sets of 10–12 reps	X	X	X

NOTES

_____

_____

_____

_____

_____

Women's Intermediate Routine · Phase 2 · Deload (Week 17)

WORKOUT 1: LOWER BODY A		
EXERCISES	**SETS** *TOTAL WEIGHT X REPS, E.G., 45 X 12*	
	SET 1	SET 2
TRAP-BAR DEADLIFT Warm-up and 2 hard sets of 8 reps	X	X
DUMBBELL LUNGE (WALKING) 2 hard sets of 8 reps	X	X
DUMBBELL ROMANIAN DEADLIFT 2 hard sets of 8 reps	X	X
DUMBBELL GOBLET SQUAT 2 hard sets of 8 reps	X	X

NOTES

_____

_____

_____

_____

_____

_____

WORKOUT 2: UPPER BODY A		
EXERCISES	**SETS** *TOTAL WEIGHT X REPS, E.G., 45 X 12*	
	SET 1	SET 2
INCLINE DUMBBELL BENCH PRESS Warm-up and 2 hard sets of 8 reps	X	X
ONE-ARM DUMBBELL ROW 2 hard sets of 8 reps	X	X

EXERCISES	SET 1	SET 2
DUMBBELL BENCH PRESS 2 hard sets of 8 reps	X	X
SEATED CABLE ROW 2 hard sets of 8 reps	X	X

NOTES

_____

_____

_____

_____

_____

WORKOUT 3: LOWER BODY B		
EXERCISES	**SETS** _TOTAL WEIGHT X REPS, E.G., 45 X 12_	
	SET 1	SET 2
DUMBBELL GOBLET SQUAT Warm-up and 2 hard sets of 8 reps	X	X
DUMBBELL DEADLIFT 2 hard sets of 8 reps	X	X
LEG EXTENSION 2 hard sets of 8 reps	X	X
LEG CURL (LYING OR SEATED) 2 hard sets of 8 reps	X	X

NOTES

_____

_____

_____

_____

_____

FOUR MONTHS OF MEN'S INTERMEDIATE WORKOUTS
Men's Intermediate Routine · Phase 2 · Week 1

WORKOUT 1: UPPER BODY A			
EXERCISES	**SETS** *TOTAL WEIGHT X REPS, E.G., 45 X 12*		
	SET 1	SET 2	SET 3
DUMBBELL BENCH PRESS Warm-up and 3 hard sets of 10–12 reps	X	X	X
LAT PULLDOWN 3 hard sets of 10–12 reps	X	X	X
MACHINE CHEST PRESS 3 hard sets of 10–12 reps	X	X	X
SEATED CABLE ROW 3 hard sets of 10–12 reps	X	X	X

NOTES

_____

_____

_____

_____

_____

WORKOUT 2: LOWER BODY A			
EXERCISES	**SETS** *TOTAL WEIGHT X REPS, E.G., 45 X 12*		
	SET 1	SET 2	SET 3
TRAP-BAR DEADLIFT Warm-up and 3 hard sets of 10–12 reps	X	X	X
DUMBBELL GOBLET SQUAT 3 hard sets of 10–12 reps	X	X	X

MICHAEL MATTHEWS

EXERCISES	SET 1	SET 2	SET 3
LEG CURL (LYING OR SEATED) 3 hard sets of 10–12 reps	X	X	X
DUMBBELL SPLIT SQUAT 3 hard sets of 10–12 reps	X	X	X

NOTES

_____

_____

_____

_____

_____

WORKOUT 3: UPPER BODY B			
EXERCISES	**SETS** _TOTAL WEIGHT X REPS, E.G., 45 X 12_		
	SET 1	**SET 2**	**SET 3**
SEATED DUMBBELL OVERHEAD PRESS Warm-up and 3 hard sets of 10–12 reps	X	X	X
SEATED CABLE ROW 3 hard sets of 10–12 reps	X	X	X
MACHINE CHEST PRESS 3 hard sets of 10–12 reps	X	X	X
ALTERNATING DUMBBELL CURL 3 hard sets of 10–12 reps	X	X	X

NOTES

_____

_____

_____

_____

_____

Men's Intermediate Routine · Phase 2 · Week 2

WORKOUT 1: UPPER BODY A			
EXERCISES	**SETS** *TOTAL WEIGHT X REPS, E.G., 45 X 12*		
	SET 1	**SET 2**	**SET 3**
DUMBBELL BENCH PRESS Warm-up and 3 hard sets of 10–12 reps	X	X	X
LAT PULLDOWN 3 hard sets of 10–12 reps	X	X	X
MACHINE CHEST PRESS 3 hard sets of 10–12 reps	X	X	X
SEATED CABLE ROW 3 hard sets of 10–12 reps	X	X	X

NOTES

_____

_____

_____

_____

_____

_____

WORKOUT 2: LOWER BODY A			
EXERCISES	**SETS** *TOTAL WEIGHT X REPS, E.G., 45 X 12*		
	SET 1	**SET 2**	**SET 3**
TRAP-BAR DEADLIFT Warm-up and 3 hard sets of 10–12 reps	X	X	X
DUMBBELL GOBLET SQUAT 3 hard sets of 10–12 reps	X	X	X

EXERCISES	SET 1	SET 2	SET 3
LEG CURL (LYING OR SEATED) 3 hard sets of 10–12 reps	X	X	X
DUMBBELL SPLIT SQUAT 3 hard sets of 10–12 reps	X	X	X

NOTES

WORKOUT 3: UPPER BODY B

EXERCISES	SETS *TOTAL WEIGHT X REPS, E.G., 45 X 12*		
	SET 1	SET 2	SET 3
SEATED DUMBBELL OVERHEAD PRESS Warm-up and 3 hard sets of 10–12 reps	X	X	X
SEATED CABLE ROW 3 hard sets of 10–12 reps	X	X	X
MACHINE CHEST PRESS 3 hard sets of 10–12 reps	X	X	X
ALTERNATING DUMBBELL CURL 3 hard sets of 10–12 reps	X	X	X

NOTES

Men's Intermediate Routine · Phase 2 · Week 3

WORKOUT 1: UPPER BODY A			
EXERCISES	**SETS** *TOTAL WEIGHT X REPS, E.G., 45 X 12*		
	SET 1	SET 2	SET 3
DUMBBELL BENCH PRESS Warm-up and 3 hard sets of 10–12 reps	X	X	X
LAT PULLDOWN 3 hard sets of 10–12 reps	X	X	X
MACHINE CHEST PRESS 3 hard sets of 10–12 reps	X	X	X
SEATED CABLE ROW 3 hard sets of 10–12 reps	X	X	X

NOTES

_____

_____

_____

_____

_____

_____

WORKOUT 2: LOWER BODY A			
EXERCISES	**SETS** *TOTAL WEIGHT X REPS, E.G., 45 X 12*		
	SET 1	SET 2	SET 3
TRAP-BAR DEADLIFT Warm-up and 3 hard sets of 10–12 reps	X	X	X
DUMBBELL GOBLET SQUAT 3 hard sets of 10–12 reps	X	X	X

EXERCISES	SET 1	SET 2	SET 3
LEG CURL (LYING OR SEATED) 3 hard sets of 10–12 reps	X	X	X
DUMBBELL SPLIT SQUAT 3 hard sets of 10–12 reps	X	X	X

NOTES

_____

_____

_____

_____

WORKOUT 3: UPPER BODY B			
EXERCISES	**SETS** _TOTAL WEIGHT X REPS, E.G., 45 X 12_		
	SET 1	SET 2	SET 3
SEATED DUMBBELL OVERHEAD PRESS Warm-up and 3 hard sets of 10–12 reps	X	X	X
SEATED CABLE ROW 3 hard sets of 10–12 reps	X	X	X
MACHINE CHEST PRESS 3 hard sets of 10–12 reps	X	X	X
ALTERNATING DUMBBELL CURL 3 hard sets of 10–12 reps	X	X	X

NOTES

_____

_____

_____

_____

Men's Intermediate Routine · Phase 2 · Week 4

WORKOUT 1: UPPER BODY A			
EXERCISES	**SETS** *TOTAL WEIGHT X REPS, E.G., 45 X 12*		
	SET 1	SET 2	SET 3
DUMBBELL BENCH PRESS Warm-up and 3 hard sets of 10–12 reps	X	X	X
LAT PULLDOWN 3 hard sets of 10–12 reps	X	X	X
MACHINE CHEST PRESS 3 hard sets of 10–12 reps	X	X	X
SEATED CABLE ROW 3 hard sets of 10–12 reps	X	X	X

NOTES

_____

_____

_____

_____

_____

_____

_____

WORKOUT 2: LOWER BODY A			
EXERCISES	**SETS** *TOTAL WEIGHT X REPS, E.G., 45 X 12*		
	SET 1	SET 2	SET 3
TRAP-BAR DEADLIFT Warm-up and 3 hard sets of 10–12 reps	X	X	X
DUMBBELL GOBLET SQUAT 3 hard sets of 10–12 reps	X	X	X

EXERCISES	SET 1	SET 2	SET 3
LEG CURL (LYING OR SEATED) 3 hard sets of 10–12 reps	X	X	X
DUMBBELL SPLIT SQUAT 3 hard sets of 10–12 reps	X	X	X

NOTES

_____

_____

_____

_____

_____

WORKOUT 3: UPPER BODY B

EXERCISES	SETS _TOTAL WEIGHT X REPS, E.G., 45 X 12_		
	SET 1	SET 2	SET 3
SEATED DUMBBELL OVERHEAD PRESS Warm-up and 3 hard sets of 10–12 reps	X	X	X
SEATED CABLE ROW 3 hard sets of 10–12 reps	X	X	X
MACHINE CHEST PRESS 3 hard sets of 10–12 reps	X	X	X
ALTERNATING DUMBBELL CURL 3 hard sets of 10–12 reps	X	X	X

NOTES

_____

_____

_____

_____

_____

Men's Intermediate Routine · Phase 2 · Week 5

WORKOUT 1: UPPER BODY A			
EXERCISES	**SETS** *TOTAL WEIGHT X REPS, E.G., 45 X 12*		
	SET 1	**SET 2**	**SET 3**
DUMBBELL BENCH PRESS Warm-up and 3 hard sets of 10–12 reps	X	X	X
LAT PULLDOWN 3 hard sets of 10–12 reps	X	X	X
MACHINE CHEST PRESS 3 hard sets of 10–12 reps	X	X	X
SEATED CABLE ROW 3 hard sets of 10–12 reps	X	X	X

NOTES

_____

_____

_____

_____

_____

_____

_____

WORKOUT 2: LOWER BODY A			
EXERCISES	**SETS** *TOTAL WEIGHT X REPS, E.G., 45 X 12*		
	SET 1	**SET 2**	**SET 3**
TRAP-BAR DEADLIFT Warm-up and 3 hard sets of 10–12 reps	X	X	X
DUMBBELL GOBLET SQUAT 3 hard sets of 10–12 reps	X	X	X

EXERCISES	SET 1	SET 2	SET 3
LEG CURL (LYING OR SEATED) 3 hard sets of 10–12 reps	X	X	X
DUMBBELL SPLIT SQUAT 3 hard sets of 10–12 reps	X	X	X

NOTES

_____

_____

_____

_____

WORKOUT 3: UPPER BODY B

EXERCISES	SETS *TOTAL WEIGHT X REPS, E.G., 45 X 12*		
	SET 1	SET 2	SET 3
SEATED DUMBBELL OVERHEAD PRESS Warm-up and 3 hard sets of 10–12 reps	X	X	X
SEATED CABLE ROW 3 hard sets of 10–12 reps	X	X	X
MACHINE CHEST PRESS 3 hard sets of 10–12 reps	X	X	X
ALTERNATING DUMBBELL CURL 3 hard sets of 10–12 reps	X	X	X

NOTES

_____

_____

_____

_____

_____

Men's Intermediate Routine · Phase 2 · Week 6

WORKOUT 1: UPPER BODY A			
EXERCISES	**SETS** *TOTAL WEIGHT X REPS, E.G., 45 X 12*		
	SET 1	SET 2	SET 3
DUMBBELL BENCH PRESS Warm-up and 3 hard sets of 10–12 reps	X	X	X
LAT PULLDOWN 3 hard sets of 10–12 reps	X	X	X
MACHINE CHEST PRESS 3 hard sets of 10–12 reps	X	X	X
SEATED CABLE ROW 3 hard sets of 10–12 reps	X	X	X

NOTES

_____

_____

_____

_____

_____

_____

WORKOUT 2: LOWER BODY A			
EXERCISES	**SETS** *TOTAL WEIGHT X REPS, E.G., 45 X 12*		
	SET 1	SET 2	SET 3
TRAP-BAR DEADLIFT Warm-up and 3 hard sets of 10–12 reps	X	X	X
DUMBBELL GOBLET SQUAT 3 hard sets of 10–12 reps	X	X	X

EXERCISES	SET 1	SET 2	SET 3
LEG CURL (LYING OR SEATED) 3 hard sets of 10–12 reps	X	X	X
DUMBBELL SPLIT SQUAT 3 hard sets of 10–12 reps	X	X	X

NOTES

_____

_____

_____

_____

_____

WORKOUT 3: UPPER BODY B

EXERCISES	SETS _TOTAL WEIGHT X REPS, E.G., 45 X 12_		
	SET 1	SET 2	SET 3
SEATED DUMBBELL OVERHEAD PRESS Warm-up and 3 hard sets of 10–12 reps	X	X	X
SEATED CABLE ROW 3 hard sets of 10–12 reps	X	X	X
MACHINE CHEST PRESS 3 hard sets of 10–12 reps	X	X	X
ALTERNATING DUMBBELL CURL 3 hard sets of 10–12 reps	X	X	X

NOTES

_____

_____

_____

_____

_____

Men's Intermediate Routine · Phase 2 · Week 7

WORKOUT 1: UPPER BODY A			
EXERCISES	**SETS** *TOTAL WEIGHT X REPS, E.G., 45 X 12*		
	SET 1	SET 2	SET 3
DUMBBELL BENCH PRESS Warm-up and 3 hard sets of 10–12 reps	X	X	X
LAT PULLDOWN 3 hard sets of 10–12 reps	X	X	X
MACHINE CHEST PRESS 3 hard sets of 10–12 reps	X	X	X
SEATED CABLE ROW 3 hard sets of 10–12 reps	X	X	X

NOTES

_____

_____

_____

_____

_____

_____

WORKOUT 2: LOWER BODY A			
EXERCISES	**SETS** *TOTAL WEIGHT X REPS, E.G., 45 X 12*		
	SET 1	SET 2	SET 3
TRAP-BAR DEADLIFT Warm-up and 3 hard sets of 10–12 reps	X	X	X
DUMBBELL GOBLET SQUAT 3 hard sets of 10–12 reps	X	X	X

EXERCISES	SET 1	SET 2	SET 3
LEG CURL (LYING OR SEATED) 3 hard sets of 10–12 reps	X	X	X
DUMBBELL SPLIT SQUAT 3 hard sets of 10–12 reps	X	X	X

NOTES

_____

_____

_____

_____

_____

WORKOUT 3: UPPER BODY B

EXERCISES	SETS _TOTAL WEIGHT X REPS, E.G., 45 X 12_		
	SET 1	SET 2	SET 3
SEATED DUMBBELL OVERHEAD PRESS Warm-up and 3 hard sets of 10–12 reps	X	X	X
SEATED CABLE ROW 3 hard sets of 10–12 reps	X	X	X
MACHINE CHEST PRESS 3 hard sets of 10–12 reps	X	X	X
ALTERNATING DUMBBELL CURL 3 hard sets of 10–12 reps	X	X	X

NOTES

_____

_____

_____

_____

_____

Men's Intermediate Routine · Phase 2 · Week 8

WORKOUT 1: UPPER BODY A			
EXERCISES	**SETS** *TOTAL WEIGHT X REPS, E.G., 45 X 12*		
	SET 1	**SET 2**	**SET 3**
DUMBBELL BENCH PRESS Warm-up and 3 hard sets of 10–12 reps	X	X	X
LAT PULLDOWN 3 hard sets of 10–12 reps	X	X	X
MACHINE CHEST PRESS 3 hard sets of 10–12 reps	X	X	X
SEATED CABLE ROW 3 hard sets of 10–12 reps	X	X	X

NOTES

_____

_____

_____

_____

_____

_____

_____

WORKOUT 2: LOWER BODY A			
EXERCISES	**SETS** *TOTAL WEIGHT X REPS, E.G., 45 X 12*		
	SET 1	**SET 2**	**SET 3**
TRAP-BAR DEADLIFT Warm-up and 3 hard sets of 10–12 reps	X	X	X
DUMBBELL GOBLET SQUAT 3 hard sets of 10–12 reps	X	X	X

EXERCISES	SET 1	SET 2	SET 3
LEG CURL (LYING OR SEATED) 3 hard sets of 10–12 reps	X	X	X
DUMBBELL SPLIT SQUAT 3 hard sets of 10–12 reps	X	X	X

NOTES

_____

_____

_____

_____

_____

WORKOUT 3: UPPER BODY B

EXERCISES	SETS *TOTAL WEIGHT X REPS, E.G., 45 X 12*		
	SET 1	SET 2	SET 3
SEATED DUMBBELL OVERHEAD PRESS Warm-up and 3 hard sets of 10–12 reps	X	X	X
SEATED CABLE ROW 3 hard sets of 10–12 reps	X	X	X
MACHINE CHEST PRESS 3 hard sets of 10–12 reps	X	X	X
ALTERNATING DUMBBELL CURL 3 hard sets of 10–12 reps	X	X	X

NOTES

_____

_____

_____

_____

_____

Men's Intermediate Routine · Phase 2 · Week 9

WORKOUT 1: UPPER BODY A			
EXERCISES	**SETS** *TOTAL WEIGHT X REPS, E.G., 45 X 12*		
	SET 1	SET 2	SET 3
INCLINE DUMBBELL BENCH PRESS Warm-up and 3 hard sets of 10–12 reps	X	X	X
LAT PULLDOWN 3 hard sets of 10–12 reps	X	X	X
MACHINE CHEST PRESS 3 hard sets of 10–12 reps	X	X	X
MACHINE ROW 3 hard sets of 10–12 reps	X	X	X

NOTES

_____

_____

_____

_____

_____

_____

WORKOUT 2: LOWER BODY A			
EXERCISES	**SETS** *TOTAL WEIGHT X REPS, E.G., 45 X 12*		
	SET 1	SET 2	SET 3
TRAP-BAR DEADLIFT Warm-up and 3 hard sets of 10–12 reps	X	X	X
DUMBBELL LUNGE (IN-PLACE) 3 hard sets of 10–12 reps	X	X	X

EXERCISES	SET 1	SET 2	SET 3
LEG CURL (LYING OR SEATED) 3 hard sets of 10–12 reps	X	X	X
LEG PRESS 3 hard sets of 10–12 reps	X	X	X

NOTES

_____

_____

_____

_____

_____

WORKOUT 3: UPPER BODY B

EXERCISES	SETS *TOTAL WEIGHT X REPS, E.G., 45 X 12*		
	SET 1	SET 2	SET 3
SEATED DUMBBELL OVERHEAD PRESS Warm-up and 3 hard sets of 10–12 reps	X	X	X
SEATED CABLE ROW 3 hard sets of 10–12 reps	X	X	X
MACHINE CHEST PRESS 3 hard sets of 10–12 reps	X	X	X
ALTERNATING DUMBBELL CURL 3 hard sets of 10–12 reps	X	X	X

NOTES

_____

_____

_____

_____

_____

Men's Intermediate Routine · Phase 2 · Week 10

WORKOUT 1: UPPER BODY A			
EXERCISES	**SETS** *TOTAL WEIGHT X REPS, E.G., 45 X 12*		
	SET 1	**SET 2**	**SET 3**
INCLINE DUMBBELL BENCH PRESS Warm-up and 3 hard sets of 10–12 reps	X	X	X
LAT PULLDOWN 3 hard sets of 10–12 reps	X	X	X
MACHINE CHEST PRESS 3 hard sets of 10–12 reps	X	X	X
MACHINE ROW 3 hard sets of 10–12 reps	X	X	X

NOTES

_____

_____

_____

_____

_____

_____

_____

WORKOUT 2: LOWER BODY A			
EXERCISES	**SETS** *TOTAL WEIGHT X REPS, E.G., 45 X 12*		
	SET 1	**SET 2**	**SET 3**
TRAP-BAR DEADLIFT Warm-up and 3 hard sets of 10–12 reps	X	X	X
DUMBBELL LUNGE (IN-PLACE) 3 hard sets of 10–12 reps	X	X	X

EXERCISES	SET 1	SET 2	SET 3
LEG CURL (LYING OR SEATED) 3 hard sets of 10–12 reps	X	X	X
LEG PRESS 3 hard sets of 10–12 reps	X	X	X

NOTES

_____

_____

_____

_____

WORKOUT 3: UPPER BODY B

EXERCISES	SETS _TOTAL WEIGHT X REPS, E.G., 45 X 12_		
	SET 1	SET 2	SET 3
SEATED DUMBBELL OVERHEAD PRESS Warm-up and 3 hard sets of 10–12 reps	X	X	X
ONE-ARM DUMBBELL ROW 3 hard sets of 10–12 reps	X	X	X
DUMBBELL BENCH PRESS 3 hard sets of 10–12 reps	X	X	X
CABLE BICEPS CURL 3 hard sets of 10–12 reps	X	X	X

NOTES

_____

_____

_____

_____

Men's Intermediate Routine · Phase 2 · Week 11

WORKOUT 1: UPPER BODY A			
EXERCISES	**SETS** TOTAL WEIGHT X REPS, E.G., 45 X 12		
	SET 1	**SET 2**	**SET 3**
INCLINE DUMBBELL BENCH PRESS Warm-up and 3 hard sets of 10–12 reps	X	X	X
LAT PULLDOWN 3 hard sets of 10–12 reps	X	X	X
MACHINE CHEST PRESS 3 hard sets of 10–12 reps	X	X	X
MACHINE ROW 3 hard sets of 10–12 reps	X	X	X

NOTES

_____
_____
_____
_____
_____
_____
_____

WORKOUT 2: LOWER BODY A			
EXERCISES	**SETS** TOTAL WEIGHT X REPS, E.G., 45 X 12		
	SET 1	**SET 2**	**SET 3**
TRAP-BAR DEADLIFT Warm-up and 3 hard sets of 10–12 reps	X	X	X
DUMBBELL LUNGE (IN-PLACE) 3 hard sets of 10–12 reps	X	X	X

EXERCISES	SET 1	SET 2	SET 3
LEG CURL (LYING OR SEATED) 3 hard sets of 10–12 reps	X	X	X
LEG PRESS 3 hard sets of 10–12 reps	X	X	X

NOTES

_____

_____

_____

_____

_____

WORKOUT 3: UPPER BODY B			
EXERCISES	**SETS** *TOTAL WEIGHT X REPS, E.G., 45 X 12*		
	SET 1	SET 2	SET 3
SEATED DUMBBELL OVERHEAD PRESS Warm-up and 3 hard sets of 10–12 reps	X	X	X
ONE-ARM DUMBBELL ROW 3 hard sets of 10–12 reps	X	X	X
DUMBBELL BENCH PRESS 3 hard sets of 10–12 reps	X	X	X
CABLE BICEPS CURL 3 hard sets of 10–12 reps	X	X	X

NOTES

_____

_____

_____

_____

_____

Men's Intermediate Routine · Phase 2 · Week 12

WORKOUT 1: UPPER BODY A			
EXERCISES	**SETS** *TOTAL WEIGHT X REPS, E.G., 45 X 12*		
	SET 1	**SET 2**	**SET 3**
INCLINE DUMBBELL BENCH PRESS Warm-up and 3 hard sets of 10–12 reps	X	X	X
LAT PULLDOWN 3 hard sets of 10–12 reps	X	X	X
MACHINE CHEST PRESS 3 hard sets of 10–12 reps	X	X	X
MACHINE ROW 3 hard sets of 10–12 reps	X	X	X

NOTES

_____

_____

_____

_____

_____

_____

WORKOUT 2: LOWER BODY A			
EXERCISES	**SETS** *TOTAL WEIGHT X REPS, E.G., 45 X 12*		
	SET 1	**SET 2**	**SET 3**
TRAP-BAR DEADLIFT Warm-up and 3 hard sets of 10–12 reps	X	X	X
DUMBBELL LUNGE (IN-PLACE) 3 hard sets of 10–12 reps	X	X	X

EXERCISES	SET 1	SET 2	SET 3
LEG CURL (LYING OR SEATED) 3 hard sets of 10–12 reps	X	X	X
LEG PRESS 3 hard sets of 10–12 reps	X	X	X

NOTES

WORKOUT 3: UPPER BODY B

EXERCISES	SETS *TOTAL WEIGHT X REPS, E.G., 45 X 12*		
	SET 1	SET 2	SET 3
SEATED DUMBBELL OVERHEAD PRESS Warm-up and 3 hard sets of 10–12 reps	X	X	X
ONE-ARM DUMBBELL ROW 3 hard sets of 10–12 reps	X	X	X
DUMBBELL BENCH PRESS 3 hard sets of 10–12 reps	X	X	X
CABLE BICEPS CURL 3 hard sets of 10–12 reps	X	X	X

NOTES

Men's Intermediate Routine · Phase 2 · Week 13

WORKOUT 1: UPPER BODY A

EXERCISES	SETS TOTAL WEIGHT X REPS, E.G., 45 X 12		
	SET 1	SET 2	SET 3
INCLINE DUMBBELL BENCH PRESS Warm-up and 3 hard sets of 10–12 reps	X	X	X
LAT PULLDOWN 3 hard sets of 10–12 reps	X	X	X
MACHINE CHEST PRESS 3 hard sets of 10–12 reps	X	X	X
MACHINE ROW 3 hard sets of 10–12 reps	X	X	X

NOTES

_____

_____

_____

_____

_____

_____

WORKOUT 2: LOWER BODY A

EXERCISES	SETS TOTAL WEIGHT X REPS, E.G., 45 X 12		
	SET 1	SET 2	SET 3
TRAP-BAR DEADLIFT Warm-up and 3 hard sets of 10–12 reps	X	X	X
DUMBBELL LUNGE (IN-PLACE) 3 hard sets of 10–12 reps	X	X	X

EXERCISES	SET 1	SET 2	SET 3
LEG CURL (LYING OR SEATED) 3 hard sets of 10–12 reps	X	X	X
LEG PRESS 3 hard sets of 10–12 reps	X	X	X

NOTES

_____

_____

_____

_____

_____

WORKOUT 3: UPPER BODY B

EXERCISES	SETS *TOTAL WEIGHT X REPS, E.G., 45 X 12*		
	SET 1	SET 2	SET 3
SEATED DUMBBELL OVERHEAD PRESS Warm-up and 3 hard sets of 10–12 reps	X	X	X
ONE-ARM DUMBBELL ROW 3 hard sets of 10–12 reps	X	X	X
DUMBBELL BENCH PRESS 3 hard sets of 10–12 reps	X	X	X
CABLE BICEPS CURL 3 hard sets of 10–12 reps	X	X	X

NOTES

_____

_____

_____

_____

_____

Men's Intermediate Routine · Phase 2 · Week 14

WORKOUT 1: UPPER BODY A			
EXERCISES	**SETS** *TOTAL WEIGHT X REPS, E.G., 45 X 12*		
	SET 1	**SET 2**	**SET 3**
INCLINE DUMBBELL BENCH PRESS Warm-up and 3 hard sets of 10–12 reps	X	X	X
LAT PULLDOWN 3 hard sets of 10–12 reps	X	X	X
MACHINE CHEST PRESS 3 hard sets of 10–12 reps	X	X	X
MACHINE ROW 3 hard sets of 10–12 reps	X	X	X

NOTES

_____

_____

_____

_____

_____

_____

WORKOUT 2: LOWER BODY A			
EXERCISES	**SETS** *TOTAL WEIGHT X REPS, E.G., 45 X 12*		
	SET 1	**SET 2**	**SET 3**
TRAP-BAR DEADLIFT Warm-up and 3 hard sets of 10–12 reps	X	X	X
DUMBBELL LUNGE (IN-PLACE) 3 hard sets of 10–12 reps	X	X	X

EXERCISES	SET 1	SET 2	SET 3
LEG CURL (LYING OR SEATED) 3 hard sets of 10–12 reps	X	X	X
LEG PRESS 3 hard sets of 10–12 reps	X	X	X

NOTES

_____

_____

_____

_____

WORKOUT 3: UPPER BODY B			
EXERCISES	**SETS** *TOTAL WEIGHT X REPS, E.G., 45 X 12*		
	SET 1	SET 2	SET 3
SEATED DUMBBELL OVERHEAD PRESS Warm-up and 3 hard sets of 10–12 reps	X	X	X
ONE-ARM DUMBBELL ROW 3 hard sets of 10–12 reps	X	X	X
DUMBBELL BENCH PRESS 3 hard sets of 10–12 reps	X	X	X
CABLE BICEPS CURL 3 hard sets of 10–12 reps	X	X	X

NOTES

_____

_____

_____

_____

Men's Intermediate Routine · Phase 2 · Week 15

WORKOUT 1: UPPER BODY A			
EXERCISES	**SETS** *TOTAL WEIGHT X REPS, E.G., 45 X 12*		
	SET 1	SET 2	SET 3
INCLINE DUMBBELL BENCH PRESS Warm-up and 3 hard sets of 10–12 reps	X	X	X
LAT PULLDOWN 3 hard sets of 10–12 reps	X	X	X
MACHINE CHEST PRESS 3 hard sets of 10–12 reps	X	X	X
MACHINE ROW 3 hard sets of 10–12 reps	X	X	X

NOTES

_____

_____

_____

_____

_____

_____

_____

WORKOUT 2: LOWER BODY A			
EXERCISES	**SETS** *TOTAL WEIGHT X REPS, E.G., 45 X 12*		
	SET 1	SET 2	SET 3
TRAP-BAR DEADLIFT Warm-up and 3 hard sets of 10–12 reps	X	X	X
DUMBBELL LUNGE (IN-PLACE) 3 hard sets of 10–12 reps	X	X	X

MICHAEL MATTHEWS

EXERCISES	SET 1	SET 2	SET 3
LEG CURL (LYING OR SEATED) 3 hard sets of 10–12 reps	X	X	X
LEG PRESS 3 hard sets of 10–12 reps	X	X	X

NOTES

_____

_____

_____

_____

_____

WORKOUT 3: UPPER BODY B			
EXERCISES	**SETS** _TOTAL WEIGHT X REPS, E.G., 45 X 12_		
	SET 1	SET 2	SET 3
SEATED DUMBBELL OVERHEAD PRESS Warm-up and 3 hard sets of 10–12 reps	X	X	X
ONE-ARM DUMBBELL ROW 3 hard sets of 10–12 reps	X	X	X
DUMBBELL BENCH PRESS 3 hard sets of 10–12 reps	X	X	X
CABLE BICEPS CURL 3 hard sets of 10–12 reps	X	X	X

NOTES

_____

_____

_____

_____

_____

Men's Intermediate Routine · Phase 2 · Week 16

WORKOUT 1: UPPER BODY A			
EXERCISES	**SETS** *TOTAL WEIGHT X REPS, E.G., 45 X 12*		
	SET 1	**SET 2**	**SET 3**
INCLINE DUMBBELL BENCH PRESS Warm-up and 3 hard sets of 10–12 reps	X	X	X
LAT PULLDOWN 3 hard sets of 10–12 reps	X	X	X
MACHINE CHEST PRESS 3 hard sets of 10–12 reps	X	X	X
MACHINE ROW 3 hard sets of 10–12 reps	X	X	X

NOTES

_____

_____

_____

_____

_____

_____

_____

WORKOUT 2: LOWER BODY A			
EXERCISES	**SETS** *TOTAL WEIGHT X REPS, E.G., 45 X 12*		
	SET 1	**SET 2**	**SET 3**
TRAP-BAR DEADLIFT Warm-up and 3 hard sets of 10–12 reps	X	X	X
DUMBBELL LUNGE (IN-PLACE) 3 hard sets of 10–12 reps	X	X	X

EXERCISES	SET 1	SET 2	SET 3
LEG CURL (LYING OR SEATED) 3 hard sets of 10–12 reps	X	X	X
LEG PRESS 3 hard sets of 10–12 reps	X	X	X

NOTES

WORKOUT 3: UPPER BODY B

EXERCISES	SETS *TOTAL WEIGHT X REPS, E.G., 45 X 12*		
	SET 1	SET 2	SET 3
SEATED DUMBBELL OVERHEAD PRESS Warm-up and 3 hard sets of 10–12 reps	X	X	X
ONE-ARM DUMBBELL ROW 3 hard sets of 10–12 reps	X	X	X
DUMBBELL BENCH PRESS 3 hard sets of 10–12 reps	X	X	X
CABLE BICEPS CURL 3 hard sets of 10–12 reps	X	X	X

NOTES

Men's Intermediate Routine · Phase 2 · Deload (Week 17)

WORKOUT 1: UPPER BODY A		
EXERCISES	**SETS** *TOTAL WEIGHT X REPS, E.G., 45 X 12*	
	SET 1	**SET 2**
INCLINE DUMBBELL BENCH PRESS Warm-up and 2 hard sets of 8 reps	X	X
LAT PULLDOWN 2 hard sets of 8 reps	X	X
MACHINE CHEST PRESS 2 hard sets of 8 reps	X	X
MACHINE ROW 2 hard sets of 8 reps	X	X

NOTES

_____

_____

_____

_____

_____

_____

WORKOUT 2: LOWER BODY A		
EXERCISES	**SETS** *TOTAL WEIGHT X REPS, E.G., 45 X 12*	
	SET 1	**SET 2**
TRAP-BAR DEADLIFT Warm-up and 2 hard sets of 8 reps	X	X
DUMBBELL LUNGE (IN-PLACE) 2 hard sets of 8 reps	X	X

EXERCISES	SET 1	SET 2
LEG CURL (LYING OR SEATED) 2 hard sets of 8 reps	X	X
LEG PRESS 2 hard sets of 8 reps	X	X

NOTES

WORKOUT 3: UPPER BODY B

EXERCISES	SETS *TOTAL WEIGHT X REPS, E.G., 45 X 12*	
	SET 1	SET 2
SEATED DUMBBELL OVERHEAD PRESS Warm-up and 2 hard sets of 8 reps	X	X
ONE-ARM DUMBBELL ROW 2 hard sets of 8 reps	X	X
DUMBBELL BENCH PRESS 2 hard sets of 8 reps	X	X
CABLE BICEPS CURL 2 hard sets of 8 reps	X	X

NOTES

CONGRATULATIONS! YOU'VE COMPLETED PHASE TWO!

I can see it now—new personal records, inches lost and gained, and a fitter, sexier you in the mirror every day. Glory be!

Your eating and exercising regimen is likely starting to feel like an integral part of your life, too, and people are probably starting to notice it. If it hasn't begun already, get ready for basically everyone you know to start asking if you're working out and what exactly you're doing.

What's more, we have another reason to revel: you've made it through the sixth month, which is significant because in my experience, if someone is going to quit, it's usually in the first three to six months. You're still here, though, and that tells me you're a breed apart and ready for Phase Three.

It might be a stretch to say it's all downhill from here, but now that you're over the six-month hump, you have the sun in your face and the wind at your back. All you have to do now is keep showing up and let momentum carry you to the promised land.

Before you jog on, however, let's do another round of reflection on how Phase Two went and how we can make Phase Three even better. Take a few minutes to mull over the following questions and write down your answers so you can easily refer back to them as needed.

1. What are three things that went particularly well in the last phase? How so?

_____

_____

_____

_____

_____

_____

_____

_____

2. What's at least one thing you could have done better? How so?

_____

_____

_____

_____

_____

3. What's at least one thing you can do to make your next phase even better than the last? To help you answer this productively, consider the following points:

- Have you been steady with your workout compliance? Or have you been habitually falling short of your plan? If the latter, consider adopting a less demanding routine. For instance, if you've been aiming for three workouts per week, you could switch to two (Upper A and Lower A), and then, later on, try the three-day routine again (or not).
- Have any exercises started to cause niggling problems like joint or muscle pains? Is it time to swap out some of them for effective alternatives that feel better? Remember, no individual exercises are mandatory for gaining muscle and strength.
- Have you noticed that progress has begun to slow down? Has this been gnawing at you? Remember that this is normal, so don't let unrealistic expectations dampen your spirits. Rather, acknowledge that progress of any kind is always praiseworthy, especially as you get older. In fact, as the years roll on, simply being able to keep training like when you were younger is a form of progress.

_____

_____

_____

_____

_____

_____

Let's also do another round of body measurements and pictures. Take the following body measurements first thing in the morning, nude, after using the bathroom and before eating or drinking anything:

DATE	WEIGHT		WAIST	CHEST
	SHOULDERS	UPPER LEGS	ARMS	CALVES

Then take flexed and unflexed pictures from the front, back, and sides. Remember to show as much skin as you feel comfortable with—the more the better—because it will give you the best idea of how your body is responding to the program (remember to put them in an individual album or folder on your phone or computer for easy reference).

Lastly, let's discuss your next training block. So long as you meet the Phase Three strength standards shared in chapter 3, continue to Phase Three of the program. If you don't meet those standards yet, however, simply repeat Phase Two, and you should get there by the end of your second round.

You can also repeat Phase Two if you just really enjoyed it or don't have access to the extra equipment required for Phase Three, but if you want to get the most out of your next training block, advance to the third and final phase of the program.

Press on!

AN UNDERRATED BENEFIT OF GETTING FIT: PEOPLE START NOTICING YOU FOR THE RIGHT REASONS.

FOUR MONTHS OF WOMEN'S ADVANCED WORKOUTS
Women's Advanced Routine · Phase 3 · Week 1

WORKOUT 1: LOWER BODY A			
EXERCISES	**SETS** *TOTAL WEIGHT X REPS, E.G., 45 X 12*		
	SET 1	SET 2	SET 3
BARBELL BACK SQUAT Warm-up and 3 hard sets of 8–10 reps	X	X	X
BARBELL DEADLIFT 3 hard sets of 8–10 reps	X	X	X
LEG CURL (LYING OR SEATED) 3 hard sets of 8–10 reps	X	X	X
DUMBBELL LUNGE (IN-PLACE) 3 hard sets of 8–10 reps	X	X	X

NOTES

_____

_____

_____

_____

_____

WORKOUT 2: UPPER BODY A			
EXERCISES	**SETS** *TOTAL WEIGHT X REPS, E.G., 45 X 12*		
	SET 1	SET 2	SET 3
BARBELL BENCH PRESS Warm-up and 3 hard sets of 8–10 reps	X	X	X
LAT PULLDOWN 3 hard sets of 8–10 reps	X	X	X

EXERCISES	SET 1	SET 2	SET 3
INCLINE BARBELL BENCH PRESS 3 hard sets of 8–10 reps	X	X	X
ONE-ARM DUMBBELL ROW 3 hard sets of 8–10 reps	X	X	X

NOTES

WORKOUT 3: LOWER BODY B

EXERCISES	SETS *TOTAL WEIGHT X REPS, E.G., 45 X 12*		
	SET 1	SET 2	SET 3
DUMBBELL LUNGE (IN-PLACE) Warm-up and 3 hard sets of 8–10 reps	X	X	X
BARBELL ROMANIAN DEADLIFT 3 hard sets of 8–10 reps	X	X	X
LEG PRESS 3 hard sets of 8–10 reps	X	X	X
CHEST DIP 3 hard sets of 8–10 reps	X	X	X

NOTES

Women's Advanced Routine · Phase 3 · Week 2

WORKOUT 1: LOWER BODY A			
EXERCISES	**SETS** TOTAL WEIGHT X REPS, E.G., 45 X 12		
	SET 1	SET 2	SET 3
BARBELL BACK SQUAT Warm-up and 3 hard sets of 8–10 reps	X	X	X
BARBELL DEADLIFT 3 hard sets of 8–10 reps	X	X	X
LEG CURL (LYING OR SEATED) 3 hard sets of 8–10 reps	X	X	X
DUMBBELL LUNGE (IN-PLACE) 3 hard sets of 8–10 reps	X	X	X

NOTES

_____

_____

_____

_____

_____

_____

WORKOUT 2: UPPER BODY A			
EXERCISES	**SETS** TOTAL WEIGHT X REPS, E.G., 45 X 12		
	SET 1	SET 2	SET 3
BARBELL BENCH PRESS Warm-up and 3 hard sets of 8–10 reps	X	X	X
LAT PULLDOWN 3 hard sets of 8–10 reps	X	X	X

EXERCISES	SET 1	SET 2	SET 3
INCLINE BARBELL BENCH PRESS 3 hard sets of 8–10 reps	X	X	X
ONE-ARM DUMBBELL ROW 3 hard sets of 8–10 reps	X	X	X

NOTES

_____

_____

_____

_____

_____

WORKOUT 3: LOWER BODY B

EXERCISES	SETS _TOTAL WEIGHT X REPS, E.G., 45 X 12_		
	SET 1	SET 2	SET 3
DUMBBELL LUNGE (IN-PLACE) Warm-up and 3 hard sets of 8–10 reps	X	X	X
BARBELL ROMANIAN DEADLIFT 3 hard sets of 8–10 reps	X	X	X
LEG PRESS 3 hard sets of 8–10 reps	X	X	X
CHEST DIP 3 hard sets of 8–10 reps	X	X	X

NOTES

_____

_____

_____

_____

Women's Advanced Routine · Phase 3 · Week 3

WORKOUT 1: LOWER BODY A

EXERCISES	SETS *TOTAL WEIGHT X REPS, E.G., 45 X 12*		
	SET 1	SET 2	SET 3
BARBELL BACK SQUAT Warm-up and 3 hard sets of 8–10 reps	X	X	X
BARBELL DEADLIFT 3 hard sets of 8–10 reps	X	X	X
LEG CURL (LYING OR SEATED) 3 hard sets of 8–10 reps	X	X	X
DUMBBELL LUNGE (IN-PLACE) 3 hard sets of 8–10 reps	X	X	X

NOTES

WORKOUT 2: UPPER BODY A

EXERCISES	SETS *TOTAL WEIGHT X REPS, E.G., 45 X 12*		
	SET 1	SET 2	SET 3
BARBELL BENCH PRESS Warm-up and 3 hard sets of 8–10 reps	X	X	X
LAT PULLDOWN 3 hard sets of 8–10 reps	X	X	X

EXERCISES	SET 1	SET 2	SET 3
INCLINE BARBELL BENCH PRESS 3 hard sets of 8–10 reps	X	X	X
ONE-ARM DUMBBELL ROW 3 hard sets of 8–10 reps	X	X	X

NOTES

WORKOUT 3: LOWER BODY B

EXERCISES	SETS *TOTAL WEIGHT X REPS, E.G., 45 X 12*		
	SET 1	SET 2	SET 3
DUMBBELL LUNGE (IN-PLACE) Warm-up and 3 hard sets of 8–10 reps	X	X	X
BARBELL ROMANIAN DEADLIFT 3 hard sets of 8–10 reps	X	X	X
LEG PRESS 3 hard sets of 8–10 reps	X	X	X
CHEST DIP 3 hard sets of 8–10 reps	X	X	X

NOTES

Women's Advanced Routine · Phase 3 · Week 4

WORKOUT 1: LOWER BODY A			
EXERCISES	**SETS** *TOTAL WEIGHT X REPS, E.G., 45 X 12*		
	SET 1	SET 2	SET 3
BARBELL BACK SQUAT Warm-up and 3 hard sets of 8–10 reps	X	X	X
BARBELL DEADLIFT 3 hard sets of 8–10 reps	X	X	X
LEG CURL (LYING OR SEATED) 3 hard sets of 8–10 reps	X	X	X
DUMBBELL LUNGE (IN-PLACE) 3 hard sets of 8–10 reps	X	X	X

NOTES

_____

_____

_____

_____

_____

_____

_____

WORKOUT 2: UPPER BODY A			
EXERCISES	**SETS** *TOTAL WEIGHT X REPS, E.G., 45 X 12*		
	SET 1	SET 2	SET 3
BARBELL BENCH PRESS Warm-up and 3 hard sets of 8–10 reps	X	X	X
LAT PULLDOWN 3 hard sets of 8–10 reps	X	X	X

MICHAEL MATTHEWS

EXERCISES	SET 1	SET 2	SET 3
INCLINE BARBELL BENCH PRESS 3 hard sets of 8–10 reps	X	X	X
ONE-ARM DUMBBELL ROW 3 hard sets of 8–10 reps	X	X	X

NOTES

WORKOUT 3: LOWER BODY B

EXERCISES	SETS *TOTAL WEIGHT X REPS, E.G., 45 X 12*		
	SET 1	SET 2	SET 3
DUMBBELL LUNGE (IN-PLACE) Warm-up and 3 hard sets of 8–10 reps	X	X	X
BARBELL ROMANIAN DEADLIFT 3 hard sets of 8–10 reps	X	X	X
LEG PRESS 3 hard sets of 8–10 reps	X	X	X
CHEST DIP 3 hard sets of 8–10 reps	X	X	X

NOTES

Women's Advanced Routine · Phase 3 · Week 5

WORKOUT 1: LOWER BODY A			
EXERCISES	**SETS** *TOTAL WEIGHT X REPS, E.G., 45 X 12*		
	SET 1	SET 2	SET 3
BARBELL BACK SQUAT Warm-up and 3 hard sets of 8–10 reps	X	X	X
BARBELL DEADLIFT 3 hard sets of 8–10 reps	X	X	X
LEG CURL (LYING OR SEATED) 3 hard sets of 8–10 reps	X	X	X
DUMBBELL LUNGE (IN-PLACE) 3 hard sets of 8–10 reps	X	X	X

NOTES

_____

_____

_____

_____

_____

_____

WORKOUT 2: UPPER BODY A			
EXERCISES	**SETS** *TOTAL WEIGHT X REPS, E.G., 45 X 12*		
	SET 1	SET 2	SET 3
BARBELL BENCH PRESS Warm-up and 3 hard sets of 8–10 reps	X	X	X
LAT PULLDOWN 3 hard sets of 8–10 reps	X	X	X

MICHAEL MATTHEWS

EXERCISES	SET 1	SET 2	SET 3
INCLINE BARBELL BENCH PRESS 3 hard sets of 8–10 reps	X	X	X
ONE-ARM DUMBBELL ROW 3 hard sets of 8–10 reps	X	X	X

NOTES

WORKOUT 3: LOWER BODY B

EXERCISES	SETS *TOTAL WEIGHT X REPS, E.G., 45 X 12*		
	SET 1	SET 2	SET 3
DUMBBELL LUNGE (IN-PLACE) Warm-up and 3 hard sets of 8–10 reps	X	X	X
BARBELL ROMANIAN DEADLIFT 3 hard sets of 8–10 reps	X	X	X
LEG PRESS 3 hard sets of 8–10 reps	X	X	X
CHEST DIP 3 hard sets of 8–10 reps	X	X	X

NOTES

Women's Advanced Routine · Phase 3 · Week 6

WORKOUT 1: LOWER BODY A

EXERCISES	SETS TOTAL WEIGHT X REPS, E.G., 45 X 12		
	SET 1	SET 2	SET 3
BARBELL BACK SQUAT Warm-up and 3 hard sets of 8–10 reps	X	X	X
BARBELL DEADLIFT 3 hard sets of 8–10 reps	X	X	X
LEG CURL (LYING OR SEATED) 3 hard sets of 8–10 reps	X	X	X
DUMBBELL LUNGE (IN-PLACE) 3 hard sets of 8–10 reps	X	X	X

NOTES

_____

_____

_____

_____

_____

_____

_____

WORKOUT 2: UPPER BODY A

EXERCISES	SETS TOTAL WEIGHT X REPS, E.G., 45 X 12		
	SET 1	SET 2	SET 3
BARBELL BENCH PRESS Warm-up and 3 hard sets of 8–10 reps	X	X	X
LAT PULLDOWN 3 hard sets of 8–10 reps	X	X	X

EXERCISES	SET 1	SET 2	SET 3
INCLINE BARBELL BENCH PRESS 3 hard sets of 8–10 reps	X	X	X
ONE-ARM DUMBBELL ROW 3 hard sets of 8–10 reps	X	X	X

NOTES

_____
_____
_____
_____

WORKOUT 3: LOWER BODY B

EXERCISES	SETS _TOTAL WEIGHT X REPS, E.G., 45 X 12_		
	SET 1	SET 2	SET 3
DUMBBELL LUNGE (IN-PLACE) Warm-up and 3 hard sets of 8–10 reps	X	X	X
BARBELL ROMANIAN DEADLIFT 3 hard sets of 8–10 reps	X	X	X
LEG PRESS 3 hard sets of 8–10 reps	X	X	X
CHEST DIP 3 hard sets of 8–10 reps	X	X	X

NOTES

_____
_____
_____
_____
_____

Women's Advanced Routine · Phase 3 · Week 7

WORKOUT 1: LOWER BODY A

EXERCISES	SETS *TOTAL WEIGHT X REPS, E.G., 45 X 12*		
	SET 1	SET 2	SET 3
BARBELL BACK SQUAT Warm-up and 3 hard sets of 8–10 reps	X	X	X
BARBELL DEADLIFT 3 hard sets of 8–10 reps	X	X	X
LEG CURL (LYING OR SEATED) 3 hard sets of 8–10 reps	X	X	X
DUMBBELL LUNGE (IN-PLACE) 3 hard sets of 8–10 reps	X	X	X

NOTES

_____

_____

_____

_____

_____

_____

_____

WORKOUT 2: UPPER BODY A

EXERCISES	SETS *TOTAL WEIGHT X REPS, E.G., 45 X 12*		
	SET 1	SET 2	SET 3
BARBELL BENCH PRESS Warm-up and 3 hard sets of 8–10 reps	X	X	X
LAT PULLDOWN 3 hard sets of 8–10 reps	X	X	X

EXERCISES	SET 1	SET 2	SET 3
INCLINE BARBELL BENCH PRESS 3 hard sets of 8–10 reps	X	X	X
ONE-ARM DUMBBELL ROW 3 hard sets of 8–10 reps	X	X	X

NOTES

_____

_____

_____

_____

_____

WORKOUT 3: LOWER BODY B			
EXERCISES	**SETS** *TOTAL WEIGHT X REPS, E.G., 45 X 12*		
	SET 1	SET 2	SET 3
DUMBBELL LUNGE (IN-PLACE) Warm-up and 3 hard sets of 8–10 reps	X	X	X
BARBELL ROMANIAN DEADLIFT 3 hard sets of 8–10 reps	X	X	X
LEG PRESS 3 hard sets of 8–10 reps	X	X	X
CHEST DIP 3 hard sets of 8–10 reps	X	X	X

NOTES

_____

_____

_____

_____

_____

Women's Advanced Routine · Phase 3 · Week 8

WORKOUT 1: LOWER BODY A			
EXERCISES	**SETS** *TOTAL WEIGHT X REPS, E.G., 45 X 12*		
	SET 1	SET 2	SET 3
BARBELL BACK SQUAT Warm-up and 3 hard sets of 8–10 reps	X	X	X
BARBELL DEADLIFT 3 hard sets of 8–10 reps	X	X	X
LEG CURL (LYING OR SEATED) 3 hard sets of 8–10 reps	X	X	X
DUMBBELL LUNGE (IN-PLACE) 3 hard sets of 8–10 reps	X	X	X

NOTES

_____

_____

_____

_____

_____

_____

_____

WORKOUT 2: UPPER BODY A			
EXERCISES	**SETS** *TOTAL WEIGHT X REPS, E.G., 45 X 12*		
	SET 1	SET 2	SET 3
BARBELL BENCH PRESS Warm-up and 3 hard sets of 8–10 reps	X	X	X
LAT PULLDOWN 3 hard sets of 8–10 reps	X	X	X

EXERCISES	SET 1	SET 2	SET 3
INCLINE BARBELL BENCH PRESS 3 hard sets of 8–10 reps	X	X	X
ONE-ARM DUMBBELL ROW 3 hard sets of 8–10 reps	X	X	X

NOTES

WORKOUT 3: LOWER BODY B

EXERCISES	SETS *TOTAL WEIGHT X REPS, E.G., 45 X 12*		
	SET 1	SET 2	SET 3
DUMBBELL LUNGE (IN-PLACE) Warm-up and 3 hard sets of 8–10 reps	X	X	X
BARBELL ROMANIAN DEADLIFT 3 hard sets of 8–10 reps	X	X	X
LEG PRESS 3 hard sets of 8–10 reps	X	X	X
CHEST DIP 3 hard sets of 8–10 reps	X	X	X

NOTES

Women's Advanced Routine · Phase 3 · Week 9

WORKOUT 1: LOWER BODY A			
EXERCISES	**SETS** *TOTAL WEIGHT X REPS, E.G., 45 X 12*		
	SET 1	**SET 2**	**SET 3**
BARBELL BACK SQUAT Warm-up and 3 hard sets of 8–10 reps	X	X	X
BARBELL ROMANIAN DEADLIFT 3 hard sets of 8–10 reps	X	X	X
LEG EXTENSION 3 hard sets of 8–10 reps	X	X	X
LEG CURL (LYING OR SEATED) 3 hard sets of 8–10 reps	X	X	X

NOTES

_____

_____

_____

_____

_____

_____

_____

WORKOUT 2: UPPER BODY A			
EXERCISES	**SETS** *TOTAL WEIGHT X REPS, E.G., 45 X 12*		
	SET 1	**SET 2**	**SET 3**
BARBELL BENCH PRESS Warm-up and 3 hard sets of 8–10 reps	X	X	X
CHIN-UP 3 hard sets of 8–10 reps	X	X	X

MICHAEL MATTHEWS

EXERCISES	SET 1	SET 2	SET 3
CHEST DIP 3 hard sets of 8–10 reps	X	X	X
SEATED CABLE ROW 3 hard sets of 8–10 reps	X	X	X

NOTES

WORKOUT 3: LOWER BODY B

EXERCISES	SETS *TOTAL WEIGHT X REPS, E.G., 45 X 12*		
	SET 1	SET 2	SET 3
BARBELL DEADLIFT Warm-up and 3 hard sets of 8–10 reps	X	X	X
DUMBBELL LUNGE (WALKING) 3 hard sets of 8–10 reps	X	X	X
INCLINE BARBELL BENCH PRESS 3 hard sets of 8–10 reps	X	X	X
LEG PRESS 3 hard sets of 8–10 reps	X	X	X

NOTES

Women's Advanced Routine · Phase 3 · Week 10

WORKOUT 1: LOWER BODY A			
EXERCISES	**SETS** *TOTAL WEIGHT X REPS, E.G., 45 X 12*		
	SET 1	SET 2	SET 3
BARBELL BACK SQUAT Warm-up and 3 hard sets of 8–10 reps	X	X	X
BARBELL ROMANIAN DEADLIFT 3 hard sets of 8–10 reps	X	X	X
LEG EXTENSION 3 hard sets of 8–10 reps	X	X	X
LEG CURL (LYING OR SEATED) 3 hard sets of 8–10 reps	X	X	X

NOTES

_____

_____

_____

_____

_____

_____

_____

WORKOUT 2: UPPER BODY A			
EXERCISES	**SETS** *TOTAL WEIGHT X REPS, E.G., 45 X 12*		
	SET 1	SET 2	SET 3
BARBELL BENCH PRESS Warm-up and 3 hard sets of 8–10 reps	X	X	X
CHIN-UP 3 hard sets of 8–10 reps	X	X	X

EXERCISES	SET 1	SET 2	SET 3
CHEST DIP 3 hard sets of 8–10 reps	X	X	X
SEATED CABLE ROW 3 hard sets of 8–10 reps	X	X	X

NOTES

_____

_____

_____

_____

_____

WORKOUT 3: LOWER BODY B			
EXERCISES	**SETS** *TOTAL WEIGHT X REPS, E.G., 45 X 12*		
	SET 1	SET 2	SET 3
BARBELL DEADLIFT Warm-up and 3 hard sets of 8–10 reps	X	X	X
DUMBBELL LUNGE (WALKING) 3 hard sets of 8–10 reps	X	X	X
INCLINE BARBELL BENCH PRESS 3 hard sets of 8–10 reps	X	X	X
LEG PRESS 3 hard sets of 8–10 reps	X	X	X

NOTES

_____

_____

_____

_____

_____

Women's Advanced Routine · Phase 3 · Week 11

WORKOUT 1: LOWER BODY A			
EXERCISES	**SETS** *TOTAL WEIGHT X REPS, E.G., 45 X 12*		
	SET 1	**SET 2**	**SET 3**
BARBELL BACK SQUAT Warm-up and 3 hard sets of 8–10 reps	X	X	X
BARBELL ROMANIAN DEADLIFT 3 hard sets of 8–10 reps	X	X	X
LEG EXTENSION 3 hard sets of 8–10 reps	X	X	X
LEG CURL (LYING OR SEATED) 3 hard sets of 8–10 reps	X	X	X

NOTES

_____

_____

_____

_____

_____

_____

_____

WORKOUT 2: UPPER BODY A			
EXERCISES	**SETS** *TOTAL WEIGHT X REPS, E.G., 45 X 12*		
	SET 1	**SET 2**	**SET 3**
BARBELL BENCH PRESS Warm-up and 3 hard sets of 8–10 reps	X	X	X
CHIN-UP 3 hard sets of 8–10 reps	X	X	X

EXERCISES	SET 1	SET 2	SET 3
CHEST DIP 3 hard sets of 8–10 reps	X	X	X
SEATED CABLE ROW 3 hard sets of 8–10 reps	X	X	X

NOTES

_____

_____

_____

_____

_____

WORKOUT 3: LOWER BODY B			
EXERCISES	**SETS** _TOTAL WEIGHT X REPS, E.G., 45 X 12_		
	SET 1	SET 2	SET 3
BARBELL DEADLIFT Warm-up and 3 hard sets of 8–10 reps	X	X	X
DUMBBELL LUNGE (WALKING) 3 hard sets of 8–10 reps	X	X	X
INCLINE BARBELL BENCH PRESS 3 hard sets of 8–10 reps	X	X	X
LEG PRESS 3 hard sets of 8–10 reps	X	X	X

NOTES

_____

_____

_____

_____

_____

Women's Advanced Routine · Phase 3 · Week 12

WORKOUT 1: LOWER BODY A

EXERCISES	SETS *TOTAL WEIGHT X REPS, E.G., 45 X 12*		
	SET 1	SET 2	SET 3
BARBELL BACK SQUAT Warm-up and 3 hard sets of 8–10 reps	X	X	X
BARBELL ROMANIAN DEADLIFT 3 hard sets of 8–10 reps	X	X	X
LEG EXTENSION 3 hard sets of 8–10 reps	X	X	X
LEG CURL (LYING OR SEATED) 3 hard sets of 8–10 reps	X	X	X

NOTES

_____

_____

_____

_____

_____

_____

WORKOUT 2: UPPER BODY A

EXERCISES	SETS *TOTAL WEIGHT X REPS, E.G., 45 X 12*		
	SET 1	SET 2	SET 3
BARBELL BENCH PRESS Warm-up and 3 hard sets of 8–10 reps	X	X	X
CHIN-UP 3 hard sets of 8–10 reps	X	X	X

EXERCISES	SET 1	SET 2	SET 3
CHEST DIP 3 hard sets of 8–10 reps	X	X	X
SEATED CABLE ROW 3 hard sets of 8–10 reps	X	X	X

NOTES

_____

_____

_____

_____

_____

WORKOUT 3: LOWER BODY B

EXERCISES	SETS *TOTAL WEIGHT X REPS, E.G., 45 X 12*		
	SET 1	SET 2	SET 3
BARBELL DEADLIFT Warm-up and 3 hard sets of 8–10 reps	X	X	X
DUMBBELL LUNGE (WALKING) 3 hard sets of 8–10 reps	X	X	X
INCLINE BARBELL BENCH PRESS 3 hard sets of 8–10 reps	X	X	X
LEG PRESS 3 hard sets of 8–10 reps	X	X	X

NOTES

_____

_____

_____

_____

Women's Advanced Routine · Phase 3 · Week 13

WORKOUT 1: LOWER BODY A

EXERCISES	SETS *TOTAL WEIGHT X REPS, E.G., 45 X 12*		
	SET 1	SET 2	SET 3
BARBELL BACK SQUAT Warm-up and 3 hard sets of 8–10 reps	X	X	X
BARBELL ROMANIAN DEADLIFT 3 hard sets of 8–10 reps	X	X	X
LEG EXTENSION 3 hard sets of 8–10 reps	X	X	X
LEG CURL (LYING OR SEATED) 3 hard sets of 8–10 reps	X	X	X

NOTES

_____

_____

_____

_____

_____

_____

WORKOUT 2: UPPER BODY A

EXERCISES	SETS *TOTAL WEIGHT X REPS, E.G., 45 X 12*		
	SET 1	SET 2	SET 3
BARBELL BENCH PRESS Warm-up and 3 hard sets of 8–10 reps	X	X	X
CHIN-UP 3 hard sets of 8–10 reps	X	X	X

EXERCISES	SET 1	SET 2	SET 3
CHEST DIP 3 hard sets of 8–10 reps	X	X	X
SEATED CABLE ROW 3 hard sets of 8–10 reps	X	X	X

NOTES

_____

_____

_____

_____

WORKOUT 3: LOWER BODY B			
EXERCISES	**SETS** _TOTAL WEIGHT X REPS, E.G., 45 X 12_		
	SET 1	SET 2	SET 3
BARBELL DEADLIFT Warm-up and 3 hard sets of 8–10 reps	X	X	X
DUMBBELL LUNGE (WALKING) 3 hard sets of 8–10 reps	X	X	X
INCLINE BARBELL BENCH PRESS 3 hard sets of 8–10 reps	X	X	X
LEG PRESS 3 hard sets of 8–10 reps	X	X	X

NOTES

_____

_____

_____

_____

Women's Advanced Routine · Phase 3 · Week 14

WORKOUT 1: LOWER BODY A			
EXERCISES	**SETS** *TOTAL WEIGHT X REPS, E.G., 45 X 12*		
	SET 1	**SET 2**	**SET 3**
BARBELL BACK SQUAT Warm-up and 3 hard sets of 8–10 reps	X	X	X
BARBELL ROMANIAN DEADLIFT 3 hard sets of 8–10 reps	X	X	X
LEG EXTENSION 3 hard sets of 8–10 reps	X	X	X
LEG CURL (LYING OR SEATED) 3 hard sets of 8–10 reps	X	X	X

NOTES

_____

_____

_____

_____

_____

_____

_____

WORKOUT 2: UPPER BODY A			
EXERCISES	**SETS** *TOTAL WEIGHT X REPS, E.G., 45 X 12*		
	SET 1	**SET 2**	**SET 3**
BARBELL BENCH PRESS Warm-up and 3 hard sets of 8–10 reps	X	X	X
CHIN-UP 3 hard sets of 8–10 reps	X	X	X

EXERCISES	SET 1	SET 2	SET 3
CHEST DIP 3 hard sets of 8–10 reps	X	X	X
SEATED CABLE ROW 3 hard sets of 8–10 reps	X	X	X

NOTES

_____

_____

_____

_____

WORKOUT 3: LOWER BODY B

EXERCISES	SETS *TOTAL WEIGHT X REPS, E.G., 45 X 12*		
	SET 1	SET 2	SET 3
BARBELL DEADLIFT Warm-up and 3 hard sets of 8–10 reps	X	X	X
DUMBBELL LUNGE (WALKING) 3 hard sets of 8–10 reps	X	X	X
INCLINE BARBELL BENCH PRESS 3 hard sets of 8–10 reps	X	X	X
LEG PRESS 3 hard sets of 8–10 reps	X	X	X

NOTES

_____

_____

_____

_____

_____

Women's Advanced Routine · Phase 3 · Week 15

WORKOUT 1: LOWER BODY A			
EXERCISES	**SETS** *TOTAL WEIGHT X REPS, E.G., 45 X 12*		
	SET 1	**SET 2**	**SET 3**
BARBELL BACK SQUAT Warm-up and 3 hard sets of 8–10 reps	X	X	X
BARBELL ROMANIAN DEADLIFT 3 hard sets of 8–10 reps	X	X	X
LEG EXTENSION 3 hard sets of 8–10 reps	X	X	X
LEG CURL (LYING OR SEATED) 3 hard sets of 8–10 reps	X	X	X

NOTES

_____

_____

_____

_____

_____

_____

_____

WORKOUT 2: UPPER BODY A			
EXERCISES	**SETS** *TOTAL WEIGHT X REPS, E.G., 45 X 12*		
	SET 1	**SET 2**	**SET 3**
BARBELL BENCH PRESS Warm-up and 3 hard sets of 8–10 reps	X	X	X
CHIN-UP 3 hard sets of 8–10 reps	X	X	X

EXERCISES	SET 1	SET 2	SET 3
CHEST DIP 3 hard sets of 8–10 reps	X	X	X
SEATED CABLE ROW 3 hard sets of 8–10 reps	X	X	X

NOTES

_____
_____
_____
_____
_____

WORKOUT 3: LOWER BODY B

EXERCISES	SETS *TOTAL WEIGHT X REPS, E.G., 45 X 12*		
	SET 1	SET 2	SET 3
BARBELL DEADLIFT Warm-up and 3 hard sets of 8–10 reps	X	X	X
DUMBBELL LUNGE (WALKING) 3 hard sets of 8–10 reps	X	X	X
INCLINE BARBELL BENCH PRESS 3 hard sets of 8–10 reps	X	X	X
LEG PRESS 3 hard sets of 8–10 reps	X	X	X

NOTES

_____
_____
_____
_____
_____

Women's Advanced Routine · Phase 3 · Week 16

WORKOUT 1: LOWER BODY A			
EXERCISES	**SETS** *TOTAL WEIGHT X REPS, E.G., 45 X 12*		
	SET 1	SET 2	SET 3
BARBELL BACK SQUAT Warm-up and 3 hard sets of 8–10 reps	X	X	X
BARBELL ROMANIAN DEADLIFT 3 hard sets of 8–10 reps	X	X	X
LEG EXTENSION 3 hard sets of 8–10 reps	X	X	X
LEG CURL (LYING OR SEATED) 3 hard sets of 8–10 reps	X	X	X

NOTES

_____

_____

_____

_____

_____

_____

_____

WORKOUT 2: UPPER BODY A			
EXERCISES	**SETS** *TOTAL WEIGHT X REPS, E.G., 45 X 12*		
	SET 1	SET 2	SET 3
BARBELL BENCH PRESS Warm-up and 3 hard sets of 8–10 reps	X	X	X
CHIN-UP 3 hard sets of 8–10 reps	X	X	X

MICHAEL MATTHEWS

EXERCISES	SET 1	SET 2	SET 3
CHEST DIP 3 hard sets of 8–10 reps	X	X	X
SEATED CABLE ROW 3 hard sets of 8–10 reps	X	X	X

NOTES

_____

_____

_____

_____

_____

WORKOUT 3: LOWER BODY B			
EXERCISES	**SETS** *TOTAL WEIGHT X REPS, E.G., 45 X 12*		
	SET 1	**SET 2**	**SET 3**
BARBELL DEADLIFT Warm-up and 3 hard sets of 8–10 reps	X	X	X
DUMBBELL LUNGE (WALKING) 3 hard sets of 8–10 reps	X	X	X
INCLINE BARBELL BENCH PRESS 3 hard sets of 8–10 reps	X	X	X
LEG PRESS 3 hard sets of 8–10 reps	X	X	X

NOTES

_____

_____

_____

_____

_____

Women's Advanced Routine · Phase 3 · Deload (Week 17)

WORKOUT 1: LOWER BODY A

EXERCISES	SETS TOTAL WEIGHT X REPS, E.G., 45 X 12	
	SET 1	SET 2
BARBELL BACK SQUAT Warm-up and 2 hard sets of 6 reps	X	X
BARBELL ROMANIAN DEADLIFT 2 hard sets of 6 reps	X	X
LEG EXTENSION 2 hard sets of 6 reps	X	X
LEG CURL (LYING OR SEATED) 2 hard sets of 6 reps	X	X

NOTES

_____

_____

_____

_____

_____

_____

WORKOUT 2: UPPER BODY A

EXERCISES	SETS TOTAL WEIGHT X REPS, E.G., 45 X 12	
	SET 1	SET 2
BARBELL BENCH PRESS Warm-up and 2 hard sets of 6 reps	X	X
CHIN-UP 2 hard sets of 6 reps	X	X

EXERCISES	SET 1	SET 2
CHEST DIP 2 hard sets of 6 reps	X	X
SEATED CABLE ROW 2 hard sets of 6 reps	X	X

NOTES

_____
_____
_____
_____
_____

WORKOUT 3: LOWER BODY B

EXERCISES	SETS _TOTAL WEIGHT X REPS, E.G., 45 X 12_	
	SET 1	SET 2
BARBELL DEADLIFT Warm-up and 2 hard sets of 6 reps	X	X
DUMBBELL LUNGE (WALKING) 2 hard sets of 6 reps	X	X
INCLINE BARBELL BENCH PRESS 2 hard sets of 6 reps	X	X
LEG PRESS 2 hard sets of 6 reps	X	X

NOTES

_____
_____
_____
_____
_____

FOUR MONTHS OF MEN'S ADVANCED WORKOUTS
Men's Advanced Routine · Phase 3 · Week 1

WORKOUT 1: UPPER BODY A			
EXERCISES	**SETS** *TOTAL WEIGHT X REPS, E.G., 45 X 12*		
	SET 1	SET 2	SET 3
BARBELL BENCH PRESS Warm-up and 3 hard sets of 8–10 reps	X	X	X
LAT PULLDOWN 3 hard sets of 8–10 reps	X	X	X
DUMBBELL BENCH PRESS 3 hard sets of 8–10 reps	X	X	X
ONE-ARM DUMBBELL ROW 3 hard sets of 8–10 reps	X	X	X

NOTES

_____

_____

_____

_____

_____

WORKOUT 2: LOWER BODY A			
EXERCISES	**SETS** *TOTAL WEIGHT X REPS, E.G., 45 X 12*		
	SET 1	SET 2	SET 3
BARBELL BACK SQUAT Warm-up and 3 hard sets of 8–10 reps	X	X	X
BARBELL DEADLIFT 3 hard sets of 8–10 reps	X	X	X

EXERCISES	SET 1	SET 2	SET 3
DUMBBELL SPLIT SQUAT 3 hard sets of 8–10 reps	X	X	X
LEG CURL (LYING OR SEATED) 3 hard sets of 8–10 reps	X	X	X

NOTES

_____

_____

_____

_____

_____

WORKOUT 3: UPPER BODY B

EXERCISES	SETS _TOTAL WEIGHT X REPS, E.G., 45 X 12_		
	SET 1	SET 2	SET 3
SEATED DUMBBELL OVERHEAD PRESS Warm-up and 3 hard sets of 8–10 reps	X	X	X
ONE-ARM DUMBBELL ROW 3 hard sets of 8–10 reps	X	X	X
DUMBBELL BENCH PRESS 3 hard sets of 8–10 reps	X	X	X
ALTERNATING DUMBBELL CURL 3 hard sets of 8–10 reps	X	X	X

NOTES

_____

_____

_____

_____

_____

Men's Advanced Routine · Phase 3 · Week 2

WORKOUT 1: UPPER BODY A			
EXERCISES	**SETS** *TOTAL WEIGHT X REPS, E.G., 45 X 12*		
	SET 1	**SET 2**	**SET 3**
BARBELL BENCH PRESS Warm-up and 3 hard sets of 8–10 reps	X	X	X
LAT PULLDOWN 3 hard sets of 8–10 reps	X	X	X
DUMBBELL BENCH PRESS 3 hard sets of 8–10 reps	X	X	X
ONE-ARM DUMBBELL ROW 3 hard sets of 8–10 reps	X	X	X

NOTES

WORKOUT 2: LOWER BODY A			
EXERCISES	**SETS** *TOTAL WEIGHT X REPS, E.G., 45 X 12*		
	SET 1	**SET 2**	**SET 3**
BARBELL BACK SQUAT Warm-up and 3 hard sets of 8–10 reps	X	X	X
BARBELL DEADLIFT 3 hard sets of 8–10 reps	X	X	X

EXERCISES	SET 1	SET 2	SET 3
DUMBBELL SPLIT SQUAT 3 hard sets of 8–10 reps	X	X	X
LEG CURL (LYING OR SEATED) 3 hard sets of 8–10 reps	X	X	X

NOTES

_____

_____

_____

_____

_____

WORKOUT 3: UPPER BODY B

EXERCISES	SETS *TOTAL WEIGHT X REPS, E.G., 45 X 12*		
	SET 1	SET 2	SET 3
SEATED DUMBBELL OVERHEAD PRESS Warm-up and 3 hard sets of 8–10 reps	X	X	X
ONE-ARM DUMBBELL ROW 3 hard sets of 8–10 reps	X	X	X
DUMBBELL BENCH PRESS 3 hard sets of 8–10 reps	X	X	X
ALTERNATING DUMBBELL CURL 3 hard sets of 8–10 reps	X	X	X

NOTES

_____

_____

_____

_____

_____

Men's Advanced Routine · Phase 3 · Week 3

WORKOUT 1: UPPER BODY A

EXERCISES	SETS *TOTAL WEIGHT X REPS, E.G., 45 X 12*		
	SET 1	SET 2	SET 3
BARBELL BENCH PRESS Warm-up and 3 hard sets of 8–10 reps	X	X	X
LAT PULLDOWN 3 hard sets of 8–10 reps	X	X	X
DUMBBELL BENCH PRESS 3 hard sets of 8–10 reps	X	X	X
ONE-ARM DUMBBELL ROW 3 hard sets of 8–10 reps	X	X	X

NOTES

_____

_____

_____

_____

_____

_____

WORKOUT 2: LOWER BODY A

EXERCISES	SETS *TOTAL WEIGHT X REPS, E.G., 45 X 12*		
	SET 1	SET 2	SET 3
BARBELL BACK SQUAT Warm-up and 3 hard sets of 8–10 reps	X	X	X
BARBELL DEADLIFT 3 hard sets of 8–10 reps	X	X	X

EXERCISES	SET 1	SET 2	SET 3
DUMBBELL SPLIT SQUAT 3 hard sets of 8–10 reps	X	X	X
LEG CURL (LYING OR SEATED) 3 hard sets of 8–10 reps	X	X	X

NOTES

WORKOUT 3: UPPER BODY B

EXERCISES	SETS *TOTAL WEIGHT X REPS, E.G., 45 X 12*		
	SET 1	SET 2	SET 3
SEATED DUMBBELL OVERHEAD PRESS Warm-up and 3 hard sets of 8–10 reps	X	X	X
ONE-ARM DUMBBELL ROW 3 hard sets of 8–10 reps	X	X	X
DUMBBELL BENCH PRESS 3 hard sets of 8–10 reps	X	X	X
ALTERNATING DUMBBELL CURL 3 hard sets of 8–10 reps	X	X	X

NOTES

Men's Advanced Routine · Phase 3 · Week 4

WORKOUT 1: UPPER BODY A			
EXERCISES	**SETS** *TOTAL WEIGHT X REPS, E.G., 45 X 12*		
	SET 1	SET 2	SET 3
BARBELL BENCH PRESS Warm-up and 3 hard sets of 8–10 reps	X	X	X
LAT PULLDOWN 3 hard sets of 8–10 reps	X	X	X
DUMBBELL BENCH PRESS 3 hard sets of 8–10 reps	X	X	X
ONE-ARM DUMBBELL ROW 3 hard sets of 8–10 reps	X	X	X

NOTES

_____

_____

_____

_____

_____

_____

_____

WORKOUT 2: LOWER BODY A			
EXERCISES	**SETS** *TOTAL WEIGHT X REPS, E.G., 45 X 12*		
	SET 1	SET 2	SET 3
BARBELL BACK SQUAT Warm-up and 3 hard sets of 8–10 reps	X	X	X
BARBELL DEADLIFT 3 hard sets of 8–10 reps	X	X	X

EXERCISES	SET 1	SET 2	SET 3
DUMBBELL SPLIT SQUAT 3 hard sets of 8–10 reps	X	X	X
LEG CURL (LYING OR SEATED) 3 hard sets of 8–10 reps	X	X	X

NOTES

_____

_____

_____

_____

_____

WORKOUT 3: UPPER BODY B

EXERCISES	SETS *TOTAL WEIGHT X REPS, E.G., 45 X 12*		
	SET 1	SET 2	SET 3
SEATED DUMBBELL OVERHEAD PRESS Warm-up and 3 hard sets of 8–10 reps	X	X	X
ONE-ARM DUMBBELL ROW 3 hard sets of 8–10 reps	X	X	X
DUMBBELL BENCH PRESS 3 hard sets of 8–10 reps	X	X	X
ALTERNATING DUMBBELL CURL 3 hard sets of 8–10 reps	X	X	X

NOTES

_____

_____

_____

_____

_____

Men's Advanced Routine · Phase 3 · Week 5

WORKOUT 1: UPPER BODY A			
EXERCISES	**SETS** *TOTAL WEIGHT X REPS, E.G., 45 X 12*		
	SET 1	**SET 2**	**SET 3**
BARBELL BENCH PRESS Warm-up and 3 hard sets of 8–10 reps	X	X	X
LAT PULLDOWN 3 hard sets of 8–10 reps	X	X	X
DUMBBELL BENCH PRESS 3 hard sets of 8–10 reps	X	X	X
ONE-ARM DUMBBELL ROW 3 hard sets of 8–10 reps	X	X	X

NOTES

_____

_____

_____

_____

_____

_____

WORKOUT 2: LOWER BODY A			
EXERCISES	**SETS** *TOTAL WEIGHT X REPS, E.G., 45 X 12*		
	SET 1	**SET 2**	**SET 3**
BARBELL BACK SQUAT Warm-up and 3 hard sets of 8–10 reps	X	X	X
BARBELL DEADLIFT 3 hard sets of 8–10 reps	X	X	X

EXERCISES	SET 1	SET 2	SET 3
DUMBBELL SPLIT SQUAT 3 hard sets of 8–10 reps	X	X	X
LEG CURL (LYING OR SEATED) 3 hard sets of 8–10 reps	X	X	X

NOTES

WORKOUT 3: UPPER BODY B

EXERCISES	SETS *TOTAL WEIGHT X REPS, E.G., 45 X 12*		
	SET 1	SET 2	SET 3
SEATED DUMBBELL OVERHEAD PRESS Warm-up and 3 hard sets of 8–10 reps	X	X	X
ONE-ARM DUMBBELL ROW 3 hard sets of 8–10 reps	X	X	X
DUMBBELL BENCH PRESS 3 hard sets of 8–10 reps	X	X	X
ALTERNATING DUMBBELL CURL 3 hard sets of 8–10 reps	X	X	X

NOTES

Men's Advanced Routine · Phase 3 · Week 6

WORKOUT 1: UPPER BODY A			
EXERCISES	**SETS** *TOTAL WEIGHT X REPS, E.G., 45 X 12*		
	SET 1	**SET 2**	**SET 3**
BARBELL BENCH PRESS Warm-up and 3 hard sets of 8–10 reps	X	X	X
LAT PULLDOWN 3 hard sets of 8–10 reps	X	X	X
DUMBBELL BENCH PRESS 3 hard sets of 8–10 reps	X	X	X
ONE-ARM DUMBBELL ROW 3 hard sets of 8–10 reps	X	X	X

NOTES

WORKOUT 2: LOWER BODY A			
EXERCISES	**SETS** *TOTAL WEIGHT X REPS, E.G., 45 X 12*		
	SET 1	**SET 2**	**SET 3**
BARBELL BACK SQUAT Warm-up and 3 hard sets of 8–10 reps	X	X	X
BARBELL DEADLIFT 3 hard sets of 8–10 reps	X	X	X

EXERCISES	SET 1	SET 2	SET 3
DUMBBELL SPLIT SQUAT 3 hard sets of 8–10 reps	X	X	X
LEG CURL (LYING OR SEATED) 3 hard sets of 8–10 reps	X	X	X

NOTES

_____

_____

_____

_____

_____

WORKOUT 3: UPPER BODY B

EXERCISES	SETS *TOTAL WEIGHT X REPS, E.G., 45 X 12*		
	SET 1	SET 2	SET 3
SEATED DUMBBELL OVERHEAD PRESS Warm-up and 3 hard sets of 8–10 reps	X	X	X
ONE-ARM DUMBBELL ROW 3 hard sets of 8–10 reps	X	X	X
DUMBBELL BENCH PRESS 3 hard sets of 8–10 reps	X	X	X
ALTERNATING DUMBBELL CURL 3 hard sets of 8–10 reps	X	X	X

NOTES

_____

_____

_____

_____

_____

Men's Advanced Routine · Phase 3 · Week 7

WORKOUT 1: UPPER BODY A			
EXERCISES	**SETS** TOTAL WEIGHT X REPS, E.G., 45 X 12		
	SET 1	**SET 2**	**SET 3**
BARBELL BENCH PRESS Warm-up and 3 hard sets of 8–10 reps	X	X	X
LAT PULLDOWN 3 hard sets of 8–10 reps	X	X	X
DUMBBELL BENCH PRESS 3 hard sets of 8–10 reps	X	X	X
ONE-ARM DUMBBELL ROW 3 hard sets of 8–10 reps	X	X	X

NOTES

_____

_____

_____

_____

_____

_____

WORKOUT 2: LOWER BODY A			
EXERCISES	**SETS** TOTAL WEIGHT X REPS, E.G., 45 X 12		
	SET 1	**SET 2**	**SET 3**
BARBELL BACK SQUAT Warm-up and 3 hard sets of 8–10 reps	X	X	X
BARBELL DEADLIFT 3 hard sets of 8–10 reps	X	X	X

EXERCISES	SET 1	SET 2	SET 3
DUMBBELL SPLIT SQUAT 3 hard sets of 8–10 reps	X	X	X
LEG CURL (LYING OR SEATED) 3 hard sets of 8–10 reps	X	X	X

NOTES

_____

_____

_____

_____

WORKOUT 3: UPPER BODY B

EXERCISES	SETS *TOTAL WEIGHT X REPS, E.G., 45 X 12*		
	SET 1	SET 2	SET 3
SEATED DUMBBELL OVERHEAD PRESS Warm-up and 3 hard sets of 8–10 reps	X	X	X
ONE-ARM DUMBBELL ROW 3 hard sets of 8–10 reps	X	X	X
DUMBBELL BENCH PRESS 3 hard sets of 8–10 reps	X	X	X
ALTERNATING DUMBBELL CURL 3 hard sets of 8–10 reps	X	X	X

NOTES

_____

_____

_____

_____

_____

Men's Advanced Routine · Phase 3 · Week 8

WORKOUT 1: UPPER BODY A			
EXERCISES	**SETS** *TOTAL WEIGHT X REPS, E.G., 45 X 12*		
	SET 1	SET 2	SET 3
BARBELL BENCH PRESS Warm-up and 3 hard sets of 8–10 reps	X	X	X
LAT PULLDOWN 3 hard sets of 8–10 reps	X	X	X
DUMBBELL BENCH PRESS 3 hard sets of 8–10 reps	X	X	X
ONE-ARM DUMBBELL ROW 3 hard sets of 8–10 reps	X	X	X

NOTES

_____

_____

_____

_____

_____

_____

_____

WORKOUT 2: LOWER BODY A			
EXERCISES	**SETS** *TOTAL WEIGHT X REPS, E.G., 45 X 12*		
	SET 1	SET 2	SET 3
BARBELL BACK SQUAT Warm-up and 3 hard sets of 8–10 reps	X	X	X
BARBELL DEADLIFT 3 hard sets of 8–10 reps	X	X	X

EXERCISES	SET 1	SET 2	SET 3
DUMBBELL SPLIT SQUAT 3 hard sets of 8–10 reps	X	X	X
LEG CURL (LYING OR SEATED) 3 hard sets of 8–10 reps	X	X	X

NOTES

_____

_____

_____

_____

_____

WORKOUT 3: UPPER BODY B

EXERCISES	SETS *TOTAL WEIGHT X REPS, E.G., 45 X 12*		
	SET 1	SET 2	SET 3
SEATED DUMBBELL OVERHEAD PRESS Warm-up and 3 hard sets of 8–10 reps	X	X	X
ONE-ARM DUMBBELL ROW 3 hard sets of 8–10 reps	X	X	X
DUMBBELL BENCH PRESS 3 hard sets of 8–10 reps	X	X	X
ALTERNATING DUMBBELL CURL 3 hard sets of 8–10 reps	X	X	X

NOTES

_____

_____

_____

_____

_____

Men's Advanced Routine · Phase 3 · Week 9

WORKOUT 1: UPPER BODY A			
EXERCISES	**SETS** *TOTAL WEIGHT X REPS, E.G., 45 X 12*		
	SET 1	SET 2	SET 3
INCLINE BARBELL BENCH PRESS Warm-up and 3 hard sets of 8–10 reps	X	X	X
CHIN-UP 3 hard sets of 8–10 reps	X	X	X
CHEST DIP 3 hard sets of 8–10 reps	X	X	X
SEATED CABLE ROW 3 hard sets of 8–10 reps	X	X	X

NOTES

_____

_____

_____

_____

_____

_____

WORKOUT 2: LOWER BODY A			
EXERCISES	**SETS** *TOTAL WEIGHT X REPS, E.G., 45 X 12*		
	SET 1	SET 2	SET 3
BARBELL BACK SQUAT Warm-up and 3 hard sets of 8–10 reps	X	X	X
BARBELL DEADLIFT 3 hard sets of 8–10 reps	X	X	X

MICHAEL MATTHEWS

EXERCISES	SET 1	SET 2	SET 3
DUMBBELL LUNGE (IN-PLACE) 3 hard sets of 8–10 reps	X	X	X
DUMBBELL ROMANIAN DEADLIFT 3 hard sets of 8–10 reps	X	X	X

NOTES

_____

_____

_____

_____

WORKOUT 3: UPPER BODY B

EXERCISES	SETS *TOTAL WEIGHT X REPS, E.G., 45 X 12*		
	SET 1	SET 2	SET 3
SEATED DUMBBELL OVERHEAD PRESS Warm-up and 3 hard sets of 8–10 reps	X	X	X
SEATED CABLE ROW 3 hard sets of 8–10 reps	X	X	X
DUMBBELL BENCH PRESS 3 hard sets of 8–10 reps	X	X	X
DUMBBELL TRICEPS OVERHEAD PRESS 3 hard sets of 8–10 reps	X	X	X

NOTES

_____

_____

_____

_____

Men's Advanced Routine · Phase 3 · Week 10

WORKOUT 1: UPPER BODY A			
EXERCISES	**SETS** *TOTAL WEIGHT X REPS, E.G., 45 X 12*		
	SET 1	SET 2	SET 3
INCLINE BARBELL BENCH PRESS Warm-up and 3 hard sets of 8–10 reps	X	X	X
CHIN-UP 3 hard sets of 8–10 reps	X	X	X
CHEST DIP 3 hard sets of 8–10 reps	X	X	X
SEATED CABLE ROW 3 hard sets of 8–10 reps	X	X	X

NOTES

_____

_____

_____

_____

_____

_____

_____

WORKOUT 2: LOWER BODY A			
EXERCISES	**SETS** *TOTAL WEIGHT X REPS, E.G., 45 X 12*		
	SET 1	SET 2	SET 3
BARBELL BACK SQUAT Warm-up and 3 hard sets of 8–10 reps	X	X	X
BARBELL DEADLIFT 3 hard sets of 8–10 reps	X	X	X

EXERCISES	SET 1	SET 2	SET 3
DUMBBELL LUNGE (IN-PLACE) 3 hard sets of 8–10 reps	X	X	X
DUMBBELL ROMANIAN DEADLIFT 3 hard sets of 8–10 reps	X	X	X

NOTES

_____

_____

_____

_____

WORKOUT 3: UPPER BODY B

EXERCISES	SETS *TOTAL WEIGHT X REPS, E.G., 45 X 12*		
	SET 1	SET 2	SET 3
SEATED DUMBBELL OVERHEAD PRESS Warm-up and 3 hard sets of 8–10 reps	X	X	X
SEATED CABLE ROW 3 hard sets of 8–10 reps	X	X	X
DUMBBELL BENCH PRESS 3 hard sets of 8–10 reps	X	X	X
DUMBBELL TRICEPS OVERHEAD PRESS 3 hard sets of 8–10 reps	X	X	X

NOTES

_____

_____

_____

_____

Men's Advanced Routine · Phase 3 · Week 11

WORKOUT 1: UPPER BODY A			
EXERCISES	**SETS** *TOTAL WEIGHT X REPS, E.G., 45 X 12*		
	SET 1	**SET 2**	**SET 3**
INCLINE BARBELL BENCH PRESS Warm-up and 3 hard sets of 8–10 reps	X	X	X
CHIN-UP 3 hard sets of 8–10 reps	X	X	X
CHEST DIP 3 hard sets of 8–10 reps	X	X	X
SEATED CABLE ROW 3 hard sets of 8–10 reps	X	X	X

NOTES

_____

_____

_____

_____

_____

_____

_____

WORKOUT 2: LOWER BODY A			
EXERCISES	**SETS** *TOTAL WEIGHT X REPS, E.G., 45 X 12*		
	SET 1	**SET 2**	**SET 3**
BARBELL BACK SQUAT Warm-up and 3 hard sets of 8–10 reps	X	X	X
BARBELL DEADLIFT 3 hard sets of 8–10 reps	X	X	X

MICHAEL MATTHEWS

EXERCISES	SET 1	SET 2	SET 3
DUMBBELL LUNGE (IN-PLACE) 3 hard sets of 8–10 reps	X	X	X
DUMBBELL ROMANIAN DEADLIFT 3 hard sets of 8–10 reps	X	X	X

NOTES

_____

_____

_____

_____

_____

WORKOUT 3: UPPER BODY B

EXERCISES	SETS *TOTAL WEIGHT X REPS, E.G., 45 X 12*		
	SET 1	SET 2	SET 3
SEATED DUMBBELL OVERHEAD PRESS Warm-up and 3 hard sets of 8–10 reps	X	X	X
SEATED CABLE ROW 3 hard sets of 8–10 reps	X	X	X
DUMBBELL BENCH PRESS 3 hard sets of 8–10 reps	X	X	X
DUMBBELL TRICEPS OVERHEAD PRESS 3 hard sets of 8–10 reps	X	X	X

NOTES

_____

_____

_____

_____

Men's Advanced Routine · Phase 3 · Week 12

WORKOUT 1: UPPER BODY A			
EXERCISES	**SETS** *TOTAL WEIGHT X REPS, E.G., 45 X 12*		
	SET 1	**SET 2**	**SET 3**
INCLINE BARBELL BENCH PRESS Warm-up and 3 hard sets of 8–10 reps	X	X	X
CHIN-UP 3 hard sets of 8–10 reps	X	X	X
CHEST DIP 3 hard sets of 8–10 reps	X	X	X
SEATED CABLE ROW 3 hard sets of 8–10 reps	X	X	X

NOTES

_____

_____

_____

_____

_____

_____

_____

WORKOUT 2: LOWER BODY A			
EXERCISES	**SETS** *TOTAL WEIGHT X REPS, E.G., 45 X 12*		
	SET 1	**SET 2**	**SET 3**
BARBELL BACK SQUAT Warm-up and 3 hard sets of 8–10 reps	X	X	X
BARBELL DEADLIFT 3 hard sets of 8–10 reps	X	X	X

EXERCISES	SET 1	SET 2	SET 3
DUMBBELL LUNGE (IN-PLACE) 3 hard sets of 8–10 reps	X	X	X
DUMBBELL ROMANIAN DEADLIFT 3 hard sets of 8–10 reps	X	X	X

NOTES

_____

_____

_____

_____

_____

WORKOUT 3: UPPER BODY B

EXERCISES	SETS _TOTAL WEIGHT X REPS, E.G., 45 X 12_		
	SET 1	SET 2	SET 3
SEATED DUMBBELL OVERHEAD PRESS Warm-up and 3 hard sets of 8–10 reps	X	X	X
SEATED CABLE ROW 3 hard sets of 8–10 reps	X	X	X
DUMBBELL BENCH PRESS 3 hard sets of 8–10 reps	X	X	X
DUMBBELL TRICEPS OVERHEAD PRESS 3 hard sets of 8–10 reps	X	X	X

NOTES

_____

_____

_____

_____

_____

Men's Advanced Routine · Phase 3 · Week 13

WORKOUT 1: UPPER BODY A

EXERCISES	SETS TOTAL WEIGHT X REPS, E.G., 45 X 12		
	SET 1	SET 2	SET 3
INCLINE BARBELL BENCH PRESS Warm-up and 3 hard sets of 8–10 reps	X	X	X
CHIN-UP 3 hard sets of 8–10 reps	X	X	X
CHEST DIP 3 hard sets of 8–10 reps	X	X	X
SEATED CABLE ROW 3 hard sets of 8–10 reps	X	X	X

NOTES

_____

_____

_____

_____

_____

_____

WORKOUT 2: LOWER BODY A

EXERCISES	SETS TOTAL WEIGHT X REPS, E.G., 45 X 12		
	SET 1	SET 2	SET 3
BARBELL BACK SQUAT Warm-up and 3 hard sets of 8–10 reps	X	X	X
BARBELL DEADLIFT 3 hard sets of 8–10 reps	X	X	X

EXERCISES	SET 1	SET 2	SET 3
DUMBBELL LUNGE (IN-PLACE) 3 hard sets of 8–10 reps	X	X	X
DUMBBELL ROMANIAN DEADLIFT 3 hard sets of 8–10 reps	X	X	X

NOTES

_____

_____

_____

_____

WORKOUT 3: UPPER BODY B

EXERCISES	SETS _TOTAL WEIGHT X REPS, E.G., 45 X 12_		
	SET 1	SET 2	SET 3
SEATED DUMBBELL OVERHEAD PRESS Warm-up and 3 hard sets of 8–10 reps	X	X	X
SEATED CABLE ROW 3 hard sets of 8–10 reps	X	X	X
DUMBBELL BENCH PRESS 3 hard sets of 8–10 reps	X	X	X
DUMBBELL TRICEPS OVERHEAD PRESS 3 hard sets of 8–10 reps	X	X	X

NOTES

_____

_____

_____

_____

Men's Advanced Routine · Phase 3 · Week 14

WORKOUT 1: UPPER BODY A

EXERCISES	SETS TOTAL WEIGHT X REPS, E.G., 45 X 12		
	SET 1	SET 2	SET 3
INCLINE BARBELL BENCH PRESS Warm-up and 3 hard sets of 8–10 reps	X	X	X
CHIN-UP 3 hard sets of 8–10 reps	X	X	X
CHEST DIP 3 hard sets of 8–10 reps	X	X	X
SEATED CABLE ROW 3 hard sets of 8–10 reps	X	X	X

NOTES

_____

_____

_____

_____

_____

_____

_____

WORKOUT 2: LOWER BODY A

EXERCISES	SETS TOTAL WEIGHT X REPS, E.G., 45 X 12		
	SET 1	SET 2	SET 3
BARBELL BACK SQUAT Warm-up and 3 hard sets of 8–10 reps	X	X	X
BARBELL DEADLIFT 3 hard sets of 8–10 reps	X	X	X

EXERCISES	SET 1	SET 2	SET 3
DUMBBELL LUNGE (IN-PLACE) 3 hard sets of 8–10 reps	X	X	X
DUMBBELL ROMANIAN DEADLIFT 3 hard sets of 8–10 reps	X	X	X

NOTES

_____

_____

_____

_____

_____

WORKOUT 3: UPPER BODY B

EXERCISES	SETS _TOTAL WEIGHT X REPS, E.G., 45 X 12_		
	SET 1	SET 2	SET 3
SEATED DUMBBELL OVERHEAD PRESS Warm-up and 3 hard sets of 8–10 reps	X	X	X
SEATED CABLE ROW 3 hard sets of 8–10 reps	X	X	X
DUMBBELL BENCH PRESS 3 hard sets of 8–10 reps	X	X	X
DUMBBELL TRICEPS OVERHEAD PRESS 3 hard sets of 8–10 reps	X	X	X

NOTES

_____

_____

_____

_____

_____

Men's Advanced Routine · Phase 3 · Week 15

WORKOUT 1: UPPER BODY A			
EXERCISES	**SETS** *TOTAL WEIGHT X REPS, E.G., 45 X 12*		
	SET 1	**SET 2**	**SET 3**
INCLINE BARBELL BENCH PRESS Warm-up and 3 hard sets of 8–10 reps	X	X	X
CHIN-UP 3 hard sets of 8–10 reps	X	X	X
CHEST DIP 3 hard sets of 8–10 reps	X	X	X
SEATED CABLE ROW 3 hard sets of 8–10 reps	X	X	X

NOTES

_____

_____

_____

_____

_____

_____

_____

WORKOUT 2: LOWER BODY A			
EXERCISES	**SETS** *TOTAL WEIGHT X REPS, E.G., 45 X 12*		
	SET 1	**SET 2**	**SET 3**
BARBELL BACK SQUAT Warm-up and 3 hard sets of 8–10 reps	X	X	X
BARBELL DEADLIFT 3 hard sets of 8–10 reps	X	X	X

EXERCISES	SET 1	SET 2	SET 3
DUMBBELL LUNGE (IN-PLACE) 3 hard sets of 8–10 reps	X	X	X
DUMBBELL ROMANIAN DEADLIFT 3 hard sets of 8–10 reps	X	X	X

NOTES

_____

_____

_____

_____

WORKOUT 3: UPPER BODY B

EXERCISES	SETS _TOTAL WEIGHT X REPS, E.G., 45 X 12_		
	SET 1	SET 2	SET 3
SEATED DUMBBELL OVERHEAD PRESS Warm-up and 3 hard sets of 8–10 reps	X	X	X
SEATED CABLE ROW 3 hard sets of 8–10 reps	X	X	X
DUMBBELL BENCH PRESS 3 hard sets of 8–10 reps	X	X	X
DUMBBELL TRICEPS OVERHEAD PRESS 3 hard sets of 8–10 reps	X	X	X

NOTES

_____

_____

_____

_____

_____

Men's Advanced Routine · Phase 3 · Week 16

WORKOUT 1: UPPER BODY A			
EXERCISES	**SETS** *TOTAL WEIGHT X REPS, E.G., 45 X 12*		
	SET 1	SET 2	SET 3
INCLINE BARBELL BENCH PRESS Warm-up and 3 hard sets of 8–10 reps	X	X	X
CHIN-UP 3 hard sets of 8–10 reps	X	X	X
CHEST DIP 3 hard sets of 8–10 reps	X	X	X
SEATED CABLE ROW 3 hard sets of 8–10 reps	X	X	X

NOTES

_____

_____

_____

_____

_____

_____

_____

WORKOUT 2: LOWER BODY A			
EXERCISES	**SETS** *TOTAL WEIGHT X REPS, E.G., 45 X 12*		
	SET 1	SET 2	SET 3
BARBELL BACK SQUAT Warm-up and 3 hard sets of 8–10 reps	X	X	X
BARBELL DEADLIFT 3 hard sets of 8–10 reps	X	X	X

EXERCISES	SET 1	SET 2	SET 3
DUMBBELL LUNGE (IN-PLACE) 3 hard sets of 8–10 reps	X	X	X
DUMBBELL ROMANIAN DEADLIFT 3 hard sets of 8–10 reps	X	X	X

NOTES

_____
_____
_____
_____
_____

WORKOUT 3: UPPER BODY B

EXERCISES	SETS _TOTAL WEIGHT X REPS, E.G., 45 X 12_		
	SET 1	SET 2	SET 3
SEATED DUMBBELL OVERHEAD PRESS Warm-up and 3 hard sets of 8–10 reps	X	X	X
SEATED CABLE ROW 3 hard sets of 8–10 reps	X	X	X
DUMBBELL BENCH PRESS 3 hard sets of 8–10 reps	X	X	X
DUMBBELL TRICEPS OVERHEAD PRESS 3 hard sets of 8–10 reps	X	X	X

NOTES

_____
_____
_____
_____
_____

Men's Advanced Routine · Phase 3 · Deload (Week 17)

WORKOUT 1: UPPER BODY A

EXERCISES	SETS *TOTAL WEIGHT X REPS, E.G., 45 X 12*	
	SET 1	SET 2
INCLINE BARBELL BENCH PRESS Warm-up and 2 hard sets of 6 reps	X	X
CHIN-UP 2 hard sets of 6 reps	X	X
CHEST DIP 2 hard sets of 6 reps	X	X
SEATED CABLE ROW 2 hard sets of 6 reps	X	X

NOTES

_____

_____

_____

_____

_____

WORKOUT 2: LOWER BODY A

EXERCISES	SETS *TOTAL WEIGHT X REPS, E.G., 45 X 12*	
	SET 1	SET 2
BARBELL BACK SQUAT Warm-up and 2 hard sets of 6 reps	X	X
BARBELL DEADLIFT 2 hard sets of 6 reps	X	X

EXERCISES	SET 1	SET 2
DUMBBELL LUNGE (IN-PLACE) 2 hard sets of 6 reps	X	X
DUMBBELL ROMANIAN DEADLIFT 2 hard sets of 6 reps	X	X

NOTES

_____

_____

_____

_____

_____

WORKOUT 3: UPPER BODY B

EXERCISES	SETS *TOTAL WEIGHT X REPS, E.G., 45 X 12*	
	SET 1	SET 2
SEATED DUMBBELL OVERHEAD PRESS Warm-up and 2 hard sets of 6 reps	X	X
SEATED CABLE ROW 2 hard sets of 6 reps	X	X
DUMBBELL BENCH PRESS 2 hard sets of 6 reps	X	X
DUMBBELL TRICEPS OVERHEAD PRESS 2 hard sets of 6 reps	X	X

NOTES

_____

_____

_____

_____

CONGRATULATIONS!
YOU'VE COMPLETED PHASE THREE!

You've done it. You've conquered Phase Three and an entire year of *Muscle for Life* training.

You've huffed and puffed, grinned and grimaced, sweated and sworn your way through more than 150 workouts, and by now you either have your best body ever or are well on your way to it. And even better, you know exactly where to go from here—more flexible dieting, more strength training, and more progress and results.

Before we continue, however, let's do something a little different to celebrate this milestone. First, record new measurements and pictures. Take the following body measurements first thing in the morning, nude, after using the bathroom and before eating or drinking anything:

DATE	WEIGHT		WAIST	CHEST
	SHOULDERS	UPPER LEGS	ARMS	CALVES

Then, take flexed and unflexed pictures from the front, back, and sides. Show as much skin as you feel comfortable with, because it'll give you the best idea of how your body is responding to the program. Then add these photos to the album or folder you set up earlier.

Now compare those measurements and pictures to those you took a year ago, before starting Phase One. How would you describe your transformation thus far? How does it make you feel? What is most significant about it to you? Take a few minutes to meditate on these questions and write down your answers so you can easily refer back to them as needed.

_____

_____

_____

_____

Also, let's examine what went well in Phase Three, what could've been better, and how you can prepare for an even better phase to follow (more on this in a moment).

1. What are three things that went particularly well in the last phase? How so?

_____

_____

_____

_____

2. What's at least one thing you could have done better? How so?

_____

_____

_____

_____

3. What's at least one thing you can do to make your next phase even better than the last?

_____

_____

_____

_____

Now, where should you go with your training from here? There are a few options worth considering:

1. YOU CAN REPEAT PHASE THREE (AS MANY TIMES AS YOU'D LIKE).

Many folks choose to do this because they're enjoying their training and making progress and thus don't care to tinker with it. If that's you, then you can simply start Phase Three of this program again and look for ways to improve the workouts based on your experience.

For example, if a workout calls for the chest dip but you find it uncomfortable, or if you prefer a variation like the machine chest press or simply want to try a new exercise, make the swap. At minimum, such changes will make your workouts more fun, and this alone can improve results.

Also, to track your workouts when repeating a phase, you can use the blank templates in the back of this book (provided for this purpose).

2. YOU CAN CREATE YOUR OWN PROGRAMMING.

If you feel ready to use everything you've learned in the last year to create your own workout routines based on your priorities and preferences, make the leap.

Before you put pen to paper, however, I suggest you read (or reread) the training section of my book *Muscle for Life* to bone up on the first principles of effective strength training. The more your workouts embrace those teachings, the more effective they'll be.

3. YOU CAN ADVANCE TO MY *BIGGER LEANER STRONGER* OR *THINNER LEANER STRONGER* PROGRAM.

If you're eager for even more challenging training (and even faster results), then you're ready for my *Bigger Leaner Stronger* (men) or *Thinner Leaner Stronger* (women) program, which you can learn about in my books by the same titles. These programs are based on many of the same training axioms you learned about in *Muscle for Life* (plus a number of additional ones) and will give you everything you need to gain much, if not most, of the muscle and strength genetically available to you.

As we come to the end of this journey together, I want to give you another round of hoots and hollers for everything you've done—I'm proud of you. You should feel accomplished, empowered, and equal to whatever you choose to tackle next in your quest for better fitness and health.

Celebrate this victory—you've earned it—and here's to many more achievements ahead!

REASON #7,899 TO GET FIT

SUDDENLY, EVEN THE MOST BASIC CLOTHING LOOKS STYLISH ON YOU.

5 FREQUENTLY ASKED QUESTIONS

> "The only man who never makes
> a mistake is the man who never
> does anything."
> —THEODORE ROOSEVELT

IF YOU HAVEN'T YET READ the companion book to this journal, *Muscle for Life*, I strongly recommend doing so. It will answer many of the most important questions you have on how to build muscle, lose fat, and get healthy, and by the end of it, you'll have everything at your fingertips to get the most out of the workouts in this journal, including how to create flexible dieting meal plans for losing fat and building muscle without starving or depriving yourself; how to use science-based supplements to improve your body composition, performance, and health; and more.

Meanwhile, in this chapter you'll find answers to commonly asked training questions that will help you avoid setbacks and stay on track on the program.

Q: CAN I DO THIS PROGRAM IF I ONLY HAVE DUMBBELLS?

A: For the most part, you're good to go. The beginner and intermediate plans are fairly easy to follow—you'll just need to change out a couple of exercises for the machines you don't have on hand and the trap-bar deadlift (if you're tackling the intermediate program). The advanced routines might need a few more tweaks since they bring more barbell moves into the mix, but it's still doable.

To help you make the right call, here's a handy chart to consult:

INSTEAD OF THE . . .	DO THE . . .
Machine Chest Press	Push-up, Dumbbell Bench Press, or Chest Dip
Trap-Bar Deadlift	Dumbbell Deadlift
Leg Curl	Dumbbell Romanian Deadlift
Lat Pulldown	Bodyweight Row
Cable Triceps Pushdown	Dumbbell Triceps Overhead Press
Leg Press	Dumbbell Goblet Squat
Seated Cable Row	One-Arm Dumbbell Row
Cable Biceps Curl	Alternating Dumbbell Curl
Machine Shoulder Press	Seated Dumbbell Overhead Press

Q: CAN I FOLLOW THIS PROGRAM IF I TRAVEL A LOT?

A: Absolutely, but you'll need to plan ahead. If you're following an intermediate or advanced strength training program, it's a big help to book hotels near decent gyms (since hotel gyms are usually middling). It's also a good idea to figure out ahead of time when you'll be hitting the weights, so you can work it into your schedule. But if neither of those options pans out, remember that any workout is better than no workout at all when you're on the road. So, do what you can, even if it's just bodyweight exercises and a bit of jogging. You can use the principles you've picked up in this book to make those sessions as effective as possible.

Q: HOW SHOULD I WARM UP FOR MY WORKOUTS?

A: The key to a proper warm-up is to warm up the muscles you'll actually be using. Jogging on the treadmill for fifteen minutes isn't going to help your dumbbell press. Dumbbell pressing will. The same goes for any other exercise. You warm up for a squat by squatting, for a press by pressing, for a row by rowing, and so on. This will help you refine your technique, reduce the risk of injury, and get more out of your hard sets.

Q: WHAT SHOULD I DO IF I CAN'T DO A SPECIFIC EXERCISE IN A WORKOUT?

A: It all depends on what's stopping you from doing the exercise.

If it's because you don't have the strength yet, switch it out for an easier exercise that you can manage. For example, if you're following one of the women's intermediate strength training routines and the trap-bar deadlift is giving you trouble, you can stick with the dumbbell deadlift until you build up the strength for the trap-bar.

If you can't do an exercise because you don't have the right gear, replace it with a similar exercise that you do have the equipment for. For instance, you can trade cable biceps curls for dumbbell curls. Just know that some exercises don't have great stand-ins. The dumbbell deadlift and goblet squat, for example, just can't match up to the barbell versions. And while the lat pulldown is similar to pull-ups and chin-ups, the latter two are much harder and unsuitable alternatives for strength training newbies (band-assisted pull-ups or chin-ups would work well, though).

To avoid substitution headaches, try not to let "equipment poverty" hold you back. A basic home gym setup or a gym membership might seem pricey, but remember—that money is a vital investment in your health and well-being, not a frivolous splurge.

If pain or physical limitations are keeping you from doing an exercise, trade it for a similar exercise that feels comfortable. Let's say you're following the men's advanced strength training routine, and the incline barbell bench press is a no-go because of an old shoulder injury. In that case, choose a comparable exercise from either the advanced or intermediate routines (the beginner exercises will be too easy for you), like the incline dumbbell bench press or machine press, which are easier on the shoulders.

Here are some common exercise replacements that work well:

IF YOU CAN'T DO THE . . .	DO THE . . .
Push-up	Incline Push-up or Knee Push-up or Wall Push-up
Chest Dip or Triceps Dip	Assisted Dip or Bench Dip or Negative Dip
Barbell Bench Press	Dumbbell Bench Press or Machine Chest Press
Incline Barbell Bench Press	Incline Dumbbell Bench Press
Pull-up	Chin-up or Assisted Pull-up or Lat Pulldown or Negative Pull-up
Barbell Deadlift	Trap-Bar Deadlift
Trap-Bar Deadlift	Dumbbell Deadlift

IF YOU CAN'T DO THE . . .	DO THE . . .
Barbell Romanian Deadlift	Dumbbell Romanian Deadlift
Barbell Back Squat	Dumbbell Goblet Squat

Q: WHAT SHOULD I DO IF I MISS OR SKIP A WORKOUT?

A: If you skip a strength training session or two in a week, you can either make them up on other days or just let them go and proceed as if you'd done them, depending on what works best for you.

If juggling your timetable around to make up for a missed session or two isn't feasible, however, don't worry about it. Skipping a workout here and there won't put a dent in your overall progress, so just let it go and carry on as usual.

But what if you miss a week or two of workouts, or even a month or more due to vacation, work, having a baby, or whatever else life wings your way? If it's only been a week or two, you should be able to jump right back in where you left off without any problems. It takes at least three to four weeks of no training for most folks to see a noticeable drop in muscle or strength.

If you've been out of the gym for several weeks or more, though, you'll need to dial back your training weights when you get back to the grind. But here's the good news: no matter how long it's been or how much progress you think you've lost, you'll get it all back fast—way faster than it took to get there the first time around.

This is largely thanks to a phenomenon called muscle memory, which refers to how muscle fibers can bounce back to their former size and strength quicker than when you first built them. Scientists are still trying to figure out exactly how this works, but it seems that strength training permanently changes the physiology of muscle cells in a way that sets them up for rapid regrowth.

So, to get back into strength training after an extended hiatus, reduce your previous training weights by . . .

- **20 percent if it's been one to two months since your last workout**
- **30 percent if it's been three to four months since your last workout**
- **50 percent if it's been five to six months since your last workout**

And before you know it, you'll be back to fighting fit.

Q: WHAT IF I HAVE TO END A WORKOUT EARLY?

A: It's all right if this happens once in a while, but try not to let it become a regular thing. If you're cutting workouts short one or more times per week for a couple of weeks straight (or a couple of weeks per month), it's time to take a hard look at your schedule and priorities and make some changes. Also, if you do end up shortening a workout, don't try to cram the missed stuff into your next session—just plow on like it never happened.

Q: IS IT A PROBLEM IF I'M NOT GETTING VERY SORE?

A: I used to believe that being sore all the time was just the price you had to pay for getting swole, like some kind of badge of honor: "Heck yeah, I have to walk down the stairs backward! My legs are gonna be massive!" I figured that the main reason we trained our muscles was to damage them, which led to soreness, so a lot of soreness must mean a lot of damage, which would lead to a lot of muscle growth, right? Not exactly.

Research shows that while muscle damage may play a role in growth, it's not a must-have. Some workouts that make you agonizingly sore can actually lead to minimal growth (like downhill running and heavy eccentric training), while others that barely make you sore at all can trigger significant hypertrophy. To make things even more confusing, the level of soreness you feel after a workout isn't a reliable way to gauge how much muscle damage you've actually done—being really sore or not very sore doesn't always match up with a high or low amount of damage.

Scientists are still trying to wrap their heads around these phenomena, but one study done by researchers at Concordia University in Montreal found that at least some of the pain we feel after a workout comes from the connective tissue that holds muscle fibers together, not from the fibers themselves. So, what we think is muscle soreness might be partly (if not mostly) connective tissue soreness.

The bottom line is, if you're not super sore after your workouts, it doesn't mean you're doing anything wrong.

Q: CAN I TRAIN MUSCLES THAT ARE STILL SORE?

A: Yes. Training sore muscles doesn't necessarily hinder recovery and prevent muscle growth. However, if you generally train too hard, you can experience chronic soreness and fatigue that compromise your performance and eventually your health. If you follow the *Muscle for Life* program as it's laid out, though, this shouldn't happen.

Q: SHOULD I ALSO DO CARDIO WITH THIS PROGRAM?

A: Yes, if you have the time (but if you don't, focus on your strength training because it pays the largest long-term health and fitness dividends).

Concurrent training (the technical term for including both cardio and strength training in your workout routine) has several unique advantages over doing just one or the other. First, as the term implies, cardio boosts the health and function of your cardiovascular system. For instance, while cardio and strength training are about equally effective for reducing blood pressure, research shows that doing both reduces blood pressure the most.

Additionally, cardio—but not strength training—helps keep your arteries flexible and responsive to changes in blood flow. Studies show that people who do the most cardio have the supplest arteries, which is crucial for maintaining healthy blood pressure levels and minimizing stress on your heart and blood vessels.

Another circulatory downside to aging is the reduction of the capillary health and density of your muscles and other tissues, and studies show that cardio can significantly increase capillary density (the number of capillaries in an area of the body) in muscle in just a few weeks.

Cardio also burns substantially more calories per unit of time than strength training does, which can help you lose fat faster and keep it off more effectively. And by combining strength training and cardio in the way I teach in *Muscle for Life*, you can maximize fat loss without hindering muscle or strength gain.

So, here's the takeaway:

With moderate, sustainable, and effective doses of strength training and cardiovascular exercise, you can build a body that looks, feels, and functions like a well-oiled machine.

Q: WILL THIS PROGRAM HELP ME LOSE WEIGHT?

A: Probably, but a better question is: Will it help you lose fat? And yes, it absolutely will. Your weight, however, may not change as much as you'd expect since strength training builds muscle, which, well, *increases* weight. What many people don't know, however, is that strength training is fantastic for losing fat (and keeping it off).

First, strength training burns more calories than you might think—about 250 to 500 calories per hour depending on how big you are and how intensely you train (the more you weigh, the more weight you lift, and the more reps you do, the more calories you burn).

Second, the muscle you gain with strength training does more than stroke your ego—it also stokes your metabolism, making it easier to lose fat and stay lean. Muscle is more metabolically active than fat, burning about 6 calories per pound per day (versus just 2 calories per pound of body fat per day), and it also costs more energy to move a heavier (more muscular) body than a lighter one.

Moreover, muscle tissue helps you maintain good metabolic health and reduce the risk of serious metabolic diseases like type 2 diabetes, obesity, and cardiovascular disease.

Third, when we train our muscles, they release particles into our blood called extracellular vesicles, which carry with them strands of genetic material called miR-1 and find their way into nearby fat cells. When miR-1 is in muscle tissue, it hinders muscle growth, but when it's in adipose tissue, it augments fat burning. So, when you do strength training, you're making your body better at both building muscle and burning fat.

All of this is why studies show the most effective exercise strategy for fat loss is a combination of cardio and strength training. And if you have to pick just one, choose the barbell over the treadmill.

6 EPILOGUE

> **"Do not regret growing older.
> It is a privilege denied to many."**
> —MARK TWAIN

MY GOAL IS TO HELP you reach your goals, and I know that if we work together as a team, we can and will succeed.

And by "work together," I mean it—I want to connect with you, keep tabs on your progress, answer any questions or address any concerns you may have, and, I hope, feature you as a success story on my website one day!

The best way to reach me is by email: mike@muscleforlife.com. I get a lot of emails every day, so it may take a week for me to get back to you, but you *will* get a reply.

I also want to invite you to join my Facebook group, which is a community of thousands of positive, supportive, like-minded people who are striving to become the best they can be, and who can answer your questions, cheer your victories, and soothe your setbacks. Here's where you can find it:

» www.muscleforlife.group

All you have to do is visit that URL and click the "+ Join Group" button, and one of my team members will approve your application.

And speaking of social media, here's where you can find me on the major networks:

- Instagram: www.instagram.com/muscleforlifefitness
- Facebook: www.facebook.com/muscleforlifefitness
- YouTube: www.youtube.com/muscleforlifefitness
- X: www.x.com/muscleforlife

If you plan on publicly announcing that you're starting *Muscle for Life*, definitely tag me and add the #muscleforlife hashtag so other people on the program can find you and follow your journey.

Thank you so much, and I hope to hear from you soon.

7

FREE BONUS MATERIAL (WORKOUTS, MEAL PLANS, AND MORE!)

> **"Don't cling to a mistake just because
> you spent a lot of time making it."**
> —AUBREY DE GREY

THANK YOU FOR CHOOSING THE *Muscle for Life Fitness Journal*. I hope you've found this journal insightful and inspiring—and most of all that it has helped you build the fit, strong body you desire.

As I mentioned at the beginning of this journal, I've provided a number of additional free resources to help you make the most of the program, including:

- All of the workouts in this journal (plus bonus workouts), neatly laid out and provided in several digital formats, including PDF, Excel, and Google Sheets
- Links to form demonstration videos for all *Muscle for Life* exercises
- Twenty *Muscle for Life* meal plans that make losing fat and gaining lean muscle as simple as possible
- My product recommendations for workout equipment, gear, and gadgets like home gym equipment, shoes, gloves, straps, and more
- A list of my favorite tools for getting and staying motivated and on track inside and outside of the gym
- A list of my all-time favorite fitness books
- And more

To get instant access to all of those free bonuses (plus a few additional surprise gifts), go here now:

» www.mfljournal.com/bonus

Repeating, extending, or modifying a workout phase? Track your training here. And if you need more tables, simply copy the format into a blank notebook (or record the same data in a note-taking app).

EXERCISES	SETS *TOTAL WEIGHT X REPS, E.G., 45 X 12*		
	SET 1	SET 2	SET 3
	X	X	X
	X	X	X
	X	X	X
	X	X	X

NOTES

_____

_____

EXERCISES	SETS *TOTAL WEIGHT X REPS, E.G., 45 X 12*		
	SET 1	SET 2	SET 3
	X	X	X
	X	X	X
	X	X	X
	X	X	X

NOTES

_____

_____

EXERCISES	SETS TOTAL WEIGHT X REPS, E.G., 45 X 12		
	SET 1	SET 2	SET 3
	X	X	X
	X	X	X
	X	X	X
	X	X	X

NOTES

_____
_____
_____
_____

EXERCISES	SETS TOTAL WEIGHT X REPS, E.G., 45 X 12		
	SET 1	SET 2	SET 3
	X	X	X
	X	X	X
	X	X	X
	X	X	X

NOTES

_____
_____
_____
_____

EXERCISES	SETS TOTAL WEIGHT X REPS, E.G., 45 X 12		
	SET 1	SET 2	SET 3
	X	X	X
	X	X	X
	X	X	X
	X	X	X

NOTES

_____

_____

_____

_____

EXERCISES	SETS TOTAL WEIGHT X REPS, E.G., 45 X 12		
	SET 1	SET 2	SET 3
	X	X	X
	X	X	X
	X	X	X
	X	X	X

NOTES

_____

_____

_____

_____

MICHAEL MATTHEWS

EXERCISES	SETS *TOTAL WEIGHT X REPS, E.G., 45 X 12*		
	SET 1	**SET 2**	**SET 3**
	X	X	X
	X	X	X
	X	X	X
	X	X	X

NOTES

_____
_____
_____
_____

EXERCISES	SETS *TOTAL WEIGHT X REPS, E.G., 45 X 12*		
	SET 1	**SET 2**	**SET 3**
	X	X	X
	X	X	X
	X	X	X
	X	X	X

NOTES

_____
_____
_____
_____

EXERCISES	SETS TOTAL WEIGHT X REPS, E.G., 45 X 12		
	SET 1	SET 2	SET 3
	X	X	X
	X	X	X
	X	X	X
	X	X	X

NOTES

_____
_____
_____
_____

EXERCISES	SETS TOTAL WEIGHT X REPS, E.G., 45 X 12		
	SET 1	SET 2	SET 3
	X	X	X
	X	X	X
	X	X	X
	X	X	X

NOTES

_____
_____
_____
_____

MICHAEL MATTHEWS

ABOUT THE AUTHOR

MICHAEL MATTHEWS is an author, podcast host, trainer, and the founder and CEO of Legion, the #1 bestselling brand of all-natural sports supplements in the world, which he started in 2014. He lives in Ocala, Florida, with his wife, their two children, and two dachshunds named Penny and Olive.